GSDF
Gluten Sugar Dairy Free

Michelle E. DeBerge

Copyright © 2015 Michelle E. DeBerge
All rights reserved.
ISBN-10: 1511527870
ISBN-13: 978-1511527873

Review

"The adventure of living the Gluten, Diary, Sugar free lifestyle is made incredibly simple in this gorgeously tasty labor of love. Michelle holds our hands and sits in the trenches right alongside us as we delve into a deeper understanding of these foods-from the history of how these GSD products have become tainted, while providing positive and scrumptious ways of doing life and lifestyle without them on our plates. Whether this is a first glimpse at the concept of the Gluten, Sugar, Dairy free lifestyle, or you have traveled this road for quite some time, Michelle artfully intertwines her personal experience and expertise to cheer us on every step of the way! Fasten your seat belts as this is the book the GSDF community has been waiting for!!!" Kate and Justin Stellman, Radio Show Hosts, Extreme Health Radio

Extreme Health Radio is a wildly popular online radio show inviting people around the globe to invest in themselves physically, spiritually and emotionally. Hosts Justin and Kate Stellman provide ever-green and life changing information from highly acclaimed doctors, scientists, healers and authors. Start your journey to discover the best version of yourself today!

http://www.extremehealthradio.com/gsdf

Dedication

I dedicate this book to my Grandmother, Barbara O'Shaughnessy. She was my "person" and always believed in me no matter what. Mistakes were forgiven, tears were wiped away, lessons were taught and no matter what, she always urged me to follow my dreams.

She understood that I had my own journey and path to follow, no matter the bends, turns or dips it took me on. She never failed to celebrate my accomplishments with me or remind me how much more I could continue to do. She urged me to always do my best, apply myself and most of believe in myself.

My Grandmother and I had a very special relationship that was more than the average Granddaughter/Grandmother bond. She was my true confidant that I shared all of my secrets, hopes, dreams and uncertainties with. I loved sending her inappropriate greeting cards that would shock most, but made her laugh.

She went over the rainbow bridge this past year, taking a piece of my heart with her. I had hoped to have my first book written before that, but I know she would be proud of me for getting this one done.

She did not always understand the "why" I did things the way I did, but she always told me to never change and that there would never be another person like me.

She loved me in the most unconditional way possible. So I dedicate this book to the memory of our true friendship and love.

Contents

Part One - What is GSDF?

1. About Gluten
2. About Dairy
3. About Sugar

Part Two - Looking at Food Differently

1. Breakfast not in a box
2. Lunch not a sandwich
3. Portable Lunches
4. Non-Sandwich Lunches

Part Three - What is Healthy Food?

1. Organic Veggies
2. What are GMO's
3. What GMO's do to the body
4. Organic Master List*
5. Non- Organic Master List*
6. Antibiotic free meat and poultry
7. Fish and Seafood

Part Four - Set Up for Success

1. My Story
2. Getting Healthy motivation
3. Understanding the triggers
4. Overcoming Cravings
5. Baby Steps to Success

Part Five - What to Have on Hand

1. Setting Up Basic Pantry
2. Setting up Basic Freezer
3. Setting up Basic Fridge

Part Six - Meals in Minutes

1. Meal Prep for the Week
2. Master Shopping List*
3. Veggie Prep
4. Salad Prep
5. Protein Prep
6. Quick Easy Flavor Profiles

Part 7: Conversions and Substitutions

Part 8: Easy Recipes

1. Asian Turkey Meatballs
2. Avocado Chocolate Mousse
3. Cashew Cream
4. Cauliflower Fried Rice
5. Cauliflower Pizza Crust
6. Chicken Divan Casserole
7. Classic Green Juice
8. Classic Pot Roast
9. Coconut Chia Seed Pudding
10. Cold Sesame Cucumber Noodles
11. Eggs in Potato Basket
12. Fennel Kale Soup
13. Garlic Shrimp
14. Gourmet Chicken Stroganoff
15. Guatemalan Black Beans
16. Hemp Seed Pesto
17. Lemon Asparagus Noodles
18. Lemony Quinoa Tabouli
19. Lentil Soup

20. Maple Dijon Chicken
21. Morning Detox Tea
22. Vegan Ranch Dressing
23. Roasted Pork Chops
24. Sautéed Spinach
25. Slow Cooker Pepper Steak
26. Stuffed Poblano Pepper
27. Sweet Potato Enchiladas
28. Tequila Orange Prawns
29. Tuscan Pork
30. Vegan Ranch Dressing
31. Veggie Herb and Egg Casserole
32. White Bean Salad
33. Zucchini Mini Muffins

Part 9: Master Lists

1. Pantry Checklist
2. Freezer Checklist
3. Fridge Checklist
4. Shopping List
5. Conversions and Substitutions

ACKNOWLEDGMENTS

I would like to acknowledge my partner for believing in me, building me the website and getting me started on my way with GSDF. Thank you for encouraging me, teaching me what I needed to know to get it done as well as for being the tester for many of the recipes. Thank you for walking by my side, guiding me, supporting me and for always being there. Without him, this book would not have come to be. Thank you for tapping into my passion, loving me enough to keep pushing me and for your constant support, help and guidance.

I would also like to acknowledge my assistant Lisa Schuck who worked long hours to help me gather the information I needed to create this book. Kept me company, was a great soundboard and encouraged me when I needed it.

I want to acknowledge my mastermind members Dr. John DeWitt and Justin Stellman who kept cheering me on and giving me advice as I created this book.

WHAT IS GSDF?

GSDF is short for Gluten, Sugar and Dairy Free. Whether you have food allergy, sensitivity or other medical condition, or you are giving up gluten, sugar and/or dairy by choice, it can be quite overwhelming knowing what is safe to eat, how to cook a different way and what to have on hand to make healthy meals. Once you learn about how toxic these ingredients are to the body, where the hidden dangers are, you will want to know how to avoid them and yet also make delicious food.

There are more food allergies today than there ever have been before. Researchers estimate that up to 15 million Americans have food allergies. This potentially deadly disease affects 1 in every 13 children. You may have even read that celebrities like Billy Bob Thornton is gluten and dairy intolerant, Robin McGraw (Dr. Phil's wife) has gluten sensitivity as does Jessica Simpson, Katherine, Duchess of Kent and many others. Some may not even be aware that they suffer from food allergies or intolerance.

One of the more common food allergies is gluten, and it has a lot to do with how wheat is grown and GMO's (or "genetically modified organisms"). Gluten can cause arthritis, joint pain, weight gain, foggy brain and more. Sugar and dairy are the causes of a lot of common illnesses today also.

Gluten Free is now posted on menus, pre-packaged food and on ready-made items. People are becoming aware of the dangers of eating it. Yet when someone is first diagnosed with a food allergy or they are removing these items for health reasons, overwhelmingly they feel limited by their food choices and do not understand how to turn old style recipes into GSDF ones.

I had to become gluten, sugar, dairy free for health reasons and at first it was a struggle. As I began to study with some of the top alternative care practitioners and began to learn how and what to eat for my health, I struggled to find recipes that were all 3: gluten, sugar and dairy free. Most recipes were normally just free of one of the ingredients. So I began to re-write my cookbooks so that all of my new recipes were GSDF.

I discovered the health benefits of herbs, juicing and found healthy ways to recreate some of my favorite dishes. Along the way I have lost over 300 pounds and am still getting healthy. I started a website that grew into a huge community where I teaches classes about being GSDF, gives cooking lessons, recipes and coaches people as they get healthy.

This book is more than an important guide how to live gluten, sugar and dairy free with ease. It discusses the health aspects of what those ingredients do to the body, how to avoid them and find the hidden dangers.

I will show you what the healthy foods are, what to have on hand for your pantry, freezer and fridge. You will be taught how to prep your meal for the week, simple meal plans and quick easy recipes. The recipes are delicious, easy to make and you will be able to create meals in minutes. I have been able to convert favorite recipes into even better tasting versions. Included inside are the GSDF Conversions and Substitutions to turn old recipes into healthy, delicious GSDF ones!

I had to write a resource that covered all the different things to easily living a healthy gluten, sugar and dairy free lifestyle because I could not find one when I began my journey. I felt that I had to go to so many different resources, learn

So many new things and was overwhelmed in the beginning. Because of that, I created this book to help you find simple solutions, quick ways to make meals, as well as have a clearer understanding of what gluten, sugar and dairy do to our bodies. I hope you enjoy the book!

I have designed an 8-week companion course to go with this book. There is so much information, tips, and ways to live GSDF that I could not fit it all in one book. This course holds your hands through the entire process and by the end you will be making delicious meal plans, have a greater understanding of toxins and hidden dangers and be set up for success.
www.glutensugardairyfree.com/companion-course

From My Kitchen Table to Yours,
Michelle E. DeBerge

About Gluten

What is gluten?

"I can't eat that. I'm on a Gluten Free Diet." This has become a pretty common phrase that we hear more and more often. In the past 10 years there has been an increase in people that cannot eat gluten. There has also been a surge in people that have no sensitivity to wheat or gluten, giving it up as well.

The word "Gluten" basically means glue. Gluten itself is the term for the proteins that exists in wheat, rye and barley and spelt. If you take some wheat flour and put water in it, that gooey feeling in your hand is the gluten. It is what puts the elastic feel in dough and makes it stretch like rubber.

For over 10,000 years we have grown wheat and our bodies were seemingly able to digest it. It was when we began to mutate the seeds to make them resistant to pests and droughts that we changed wheat. A blend of genetic mutation and chemical use has caused modern day wheat to be bad for the body.

"We have mutant seeds, grown in synthetic soil, bathed in chemicals. They're deconstructed, pulverized to fine dust, bleached and chemically treated to create a barren industrial filler that no other creature on the planet will eat. And we wonder why it might be making us sick?"

-David Zivot, Founder GrainStorm

What does gluten do to the body?

Gluten's inflammatory effect in the gut causes intestinal cells to die prematurely and causes oxidation of those cells. Oxidation damages the cell membranes and causes "free radicals" which steal electrons from other cells. This is how the body can get disease.

"Nearly twenty million people contend that they regularly experience distress after eating products that contain gluten, and a third of American adults say that they are trying to eliminate it from their diets." Michael Specter, The New Yorker

There are more food allergies today than there ever have been before. Researchers estimate that up to 15 million Americans have food allergies. This potentially deadly disease affects 1 in every 13 children. You may have even read that celebrities like Billy Bob Thornton is gluten and dairy intolerant, Robin McGraw (Dr. Phil's wife) has gluten sensitivity as does Jessica Simpson, Katherine, Duchess of Kent and many others

From movie stars, Olympic athletes, NFL football players, musicians and so many other people suffer from gluten intolerance. Some may not even be aware that they do.

David Perlmutter, a neurologist and the author of Grain Brain: The Surprising Truth About Wheat, Carbs, and Sugar—Your Brain's Silent Killers," writes that Gluten sensitivity: "represents one of the greatest and most under-recognized health threats to humanity."

Michael Specter, The New Yorker, wrote: "Peter Gibson, a professor of gastroenterology at Monash University and the director of the G.I. unit at the Alfred Hospital, in Melbourne, seemed to provide evidence that gluten was capable of causing illness even in people who did not have celiac disease."

One of the more common food allergies is gluten, and it has a lot to do with how wheat is grown and GMO's (or "genetically modified organisms").
Gluten can cause arthritis, joint pain, weight gain, foggy brain and more.

"Gluten causes gut inflammation in at least 80% of the population and another 30% of the population develops antibodies against gluten proteins in the gut. Furthermore, 99% of the population has the genetic potential to develop antibodies against gluten." Sébastien Noël

Gluten's inflammatory effect in the gut causes intestinal cells to die prematurely and causes oxidation of those cells. This effect creates a leaky gut, which can lead to many health problems.

Leaky Gut

Leaky Gut Syndrome is another way to describe "Hyperpermeable Intestines". This is when the intestinal lining has holes developing inside of it, hence becoming more porous. When this happens the intestines cannot do their job to screen things from entering your bloodstream. A healthy intestines job is to make sure that toxins like undigested food, waste or yeast does not get into the bloodstream. A leaky gut cannot do that and toxins flow out of your intestines into the bloodstream and it causes illness.

You can become deficient in nutrients, have headaches, foggy brain, memory loss, excessive fatigue, digestive issues, lower immune system, inflammation, muscle pain, toxin build up and get yeast overgrowth called Candida which then can lead to very serious medical conditions. All because your bloodstream is now full of foreign objects that your gut can no longer filter out for you.

In fact a leaky gut affects the whole body, including the brain, which can lead to depression, anxiety, migraines and autism. One of the first steps to healing a leaky gut is to remove gluten from the diet.

Hidden dangers

Gluten can hide in many places that you may not expect like dextrin's, diglycerides, emulsifiers, enzymes, fat replacers and flavorings to list a few. Many beauty products contain gluten, as do some vitamins and medications. Once you become familiar with where gluten hides, the more you will be able to avoid it.

- Soy sauce

- Lunch meats

- Malt vinegar

- Flavorings

- Food starch

- Beauty products

- Some vitamins

- Some medications

Substitutions

The most common place that we think that gluten will appear is in is bread. Knowing that to be gluten free means to give up bread, as we know it. It does not mean that there are not wonderful substitutions available, such as from gluten free breads, rolls and flour, which are now available.

Here are some basic substitutions for items that have gluten:

Flour- use coconut flour, almond flour, amaranth flour

Bread- bread made from tapioca or rice as well as the flours above

Pasta- pasta made from rice, corn or quinoa

Soy Sauce- use coconut aminos or tamarind sauce

About Sugar

What is Sugar?

Wikipedia defines sugar as "the generalized name for sweet, short-chain, soluble carbohydrates, many of which are used in food. They are carbohydrates, composed of carbon, hydrogen, and oxygen. There are various types of sugar derived from different sources."

There are 3 main types of sugars: Sucrose, maltose, and lactose. Sucrose is the type of sugar that comes from sugar cane, beets and carrots. Maltose is the type of sugar that forms in the germination of grains. Like when barley is being turned into malt. Lactose is a natural form of sugar found in milk. All three types of these natural sugars are found in fruits and vegetables.

The sugar that is bad for the human body is the refined sugar that is chemically processed to remove the molasses from it. Molasses is the bi-product of refining sugar.

Toxins in Sugar

"Dr. David Reuben, author of Everything You Always Wanted to Know About Nutrition says, "White refined sugar-is not a food. It is a pure chemical extracted from plant sources, purer in fact than cocaine, which it resembles in many ways. Its true name is sucrose and its chemical formula is $C_{12}H_{22}O_{11}$. It has 12 carbon atoms, 22 hydrogen atoms, 11 oxygen atoms, and absolutely nothing else to offer." "...The chemical formula for cocaine is $C_{17}H_{21}NO_4$. Sugar's formula again is $C_{12}H_{22}O_{11}$. For all practical purposes, the difference is that sugar is missing the "N", or nitrogen atom."

According to the Macrobiotic Guide, "During the refining process, 64 food elements are destroyed. All the potassium, magnesium, calcium, iron, manganese, phosphate, and sulfate are removed. The A, D, and B, vitamins are destroyed. Amino acids, vital enzymes, unsaturated fats, and all fiber are gone. To a lesser or greater degree, all refined sweeteners such as corn syrup, maple syrup, etc., undergo similar destructive processes."

What it does to the body

According to the Macrobiotic Guide, "refined sugar contains no fiber, no minerals, no proteins, no fats, no enzymes, only empty calories. What happens when you eat a refined carbohydrate like sugar? Your body must borrow vital nutrients from healthy cells to metabolize the incomplete food. Calcium, sodium, potassium and magnesium are taken from various parts of the body to make use of the sugar. Refined sugar is void of all nutrients, consequently it causes the body to deplete its own stores of various vitamins, minerals and enzymes."

"As it pertains to leaky gut, you should know that sugar, like grains, can upset the balance of bacteria in your digestive tract, encouraging damage to your intestinal lining that can lead to leaky gut. So, sugary children's cereals are a double-edged sword, assaulting your fragile gastrointestinal tract with both damaging sugar and grains."

"One of the most recent studies, reported in TIME Magazine last year, found that consuming added sugars raises the risk for heart disease by raising cholesterol and triglycerides. The American Heart Association's (AHA) Web site states, "High intake of added sugars is implicated in numerous poor health conditions, including obesity, high blood pressure and other risk factors for heart disease and stroke." Dr.Mercola, Ultimate Wellness Game Changer

"Artificial sugars/sweeteners that are made in such a way that the body cannot digest them which is why they don't provide any calories. However, the bacteria in your gut can digest them, and will subsequently flourish, causing diarrhea and gas etc. A bit similar to lactose." Dr. Marije Hamaker,

Where it hides

Sugar can be hidden in many places like tomato sauce, peanut butter, salad dressings, yogurt, canned soup, canned veggies, bbq sauce, marinades and breads. [See previous comment on examples and lists]

- Tomato sauce
- Peanut Butter
- Salad Dressings
- Yogurt
- Canned Soup
- Canned Veggies
- Marinades

Healthy Sugars

Naturally contained sugars which are contained in fruit and vegetables are balanced by the fiber, vitamins, enzymes as well as the other properties of the fruit or vegetable.

Some healthy sugars that you might want to consider using are coconut sugar, raw honey and pure maple syrup.

About Dairy

"Lactose is the most common intolerance. An estimated three out of every ten Americans adults—particularly people of African, Asian, or Mediterranean heritage—don't produce enough of the enzyme lactase to digest all the lactose (milk sugar) they consume. When too much undigested lactose reaches the large intestine, it can cause gas or diarrhea." David Schardt, Nutrition Action

What is Dairy?

Dairy is a food produced from the milk of mammals. All foods derived from or containing milk that retain their calcium content are considered dairy. This includes milk, butter, yogurt and all cheese -- hard, soft and cream. Even a small amount of dairy in a food can cause the food to be considered dairy. Even things like calcium fortified juice or soymilk is considered dairy.

What dairy does to the body?

According to Dr. Oz: "The dairy in your diet could actually be causing health problems like weight gain, heartburn, lack of energy, high cholesterol, joint pain, lactose intolerance, and even irritable bowel syndrome."

"There are special lactoferrins and immunoglobulin's in dairy that is cow-specific immunizing stuff that in humans serve as allergens. The protein lactalbumin, which has been identified as a key factor in diabetes is in cow's milk. "

75 percent of the world's population is genetically unable to properly digest milk and other dairy products. By ingesting dairy, it can cause humans to have allergies, diabetes, put toxins in the bloodstream and even cause cancer. It also adds to obesity and many other illnesses.

Karen Kaplan wrote in the LA Times that a study in the journal BMJ that tracked more than 100,000 Swedish men and women for 23 years found that the avid milk drinkers were more likely to die at younger ages than their counterparts who drank little to no milk.

"D-galactose, this is produced by the body as it breaks down lactose, the sugar in milk. Studies in animals have shown that chronic exposure to the nutrient causes "oxidative stress damage, chronic inflammation, neurodegeneration, decreased immune response, and gene transcriptional changes," they wrote. In fact, when scientists want to mimic the effects of aging, they give animals shots or food containing D-galactose." The research Team from Uppsala University

The Boston Globe has described Dr. Willett as "the world's most influential nutritionist," a quiet-spoken physician and academic. According to Dr. Willett, who has done many studies and reviewed the research on this topic, there are many reasons to pass up milk, including:

Milk doesn't reduce fractures. Contrary to popular belief, eating dairy products has never been shown to reduce fracture risk. In fact, according to the Nurses' Health Study dairy may increase risk of fractures by 50 percent! Less dairy actually creates better bones. Countries with lowest rates of dairy and calcium consumption (like those in Africa and Asia) have the lowest rates of osteoporosis.

Calcium may raise cancer risk. Research shows that higher intakes of both calcium and dairy products may increase a man's risk of prostate cancer by 30 to 50 percent. 75 percent of the world's population is genetically unable to properly digest milk and other dairy products.

Toxins in Dairy

Cows milk is perfect for the calf until it is weaned and it is toxic to the human body for many reasons. According to David Reitz, cow's milk, both regular and organic milk has 59 active hormones.

Most cows' milk has measurable quantities of herbicides, pesticides, up to 52 powerful antibiotics, blood, pus, feces, bacteria and viruses. All of this can get ingested into your body.

A lot of the reasons why milk is toxic are due to what is being done to cows to have them producing milk longer than the calf needs so that humans can consume it. One of the problems is that the milk has a powerful growth hormone, IGF-1. Both cows and humans make this growth hormone. It is good for the calves that need to grow or for humans who have that hormone in their milk for their babies. Yet when we continue to ingest this hormone, it can actually lead to toxins that can cause cancer.

Cows are also given chemical injections to force them to produce more milk than naturally and these chemicals get into the milk, humans ingest it and it gets into the bloodstream where it can cause serious illness and even cancer.

Cow's milk can also have traces of anything the cow ate, including such things as radioactive fallout from nuclear testing, feces, insects or disease.

Hidden dangers and places of dairy

Dairy and dairy products are hidden in products that you might not expect like breath mints, candy, canned tuna fish, tubes of herbs, gum, some chicken broths, fat replacers, certain medications, vitamins, fried foods, protein powders, salad dressings, lunch meats, many soy products and spice mixes to name a few. Even many lactose free milks, these will still be loaded with milk proteins.

- Breath mints

- Candy

- Canned tuna fish

- Tubes of herbs

- Gum

- Some chicken stock

- Protein powders

- Salad Dressings

- Lunch Meats

Substitutions

Here are some basic substitutions for items that have dairy:

One cup cow's milk: use one cup of the following: soy milk (plain), rice milk, fruit juice, water, coconut milk or hemp milk.

One cup of yogurt: use one cup of the following: coconut yogurt, soy sour cream, unsweetened applesauce or fruit puree.

One stick of butter: use one of the following:
- 8 tablespoons of coconut oil
- 8 tablespoons Earth Balance (Non-Dairy) Buttery Spread, or other vegan substitute
- 8 tablespoons Vegan Organic Shortening
- 8 tablespoons vegetable or olive oil
- 6 tablespoons unsweetened applesauce + 2 tablespoons on of the others in this list.

Take our 8-week companion course and master all of these topics with personal support and help. The course gives you more tools that you can use in your daily life with ease. www.glutensugardairyfree.com/companion-course

Looking at Food Differently

One of the first things to do when living gluten, sugar, dairy free is to start looking at food differently than you have in the past. Fast food and ready-made options are not the best choices since most of them have hidden gluten, sugar and/or dairy in them.

Pre-packaged food showed up on the scene in 1944 when William Maxoms frozen meals showed up on airlines. In 1952 Quaker Foods started selling frozen dinners. These were the first frozen dinners that were served on aluminum trays that would heat in the home oven. Later Swanson's started marketing these frozen dinners as "TV Dinners" and they grew in popularity.

In the 1930's a surplus of molasses brought about the invention of cake mixes. The first one was a mix for gingerbread. Soon after frozen meals and pre-packaged food became the norm.

The first fast food chains originated in the United States. The first fast food chain A & W opened in 1919 and White Castle in 1921. Now there are fast food chains around the world.

As lives got busier and food got easier to grab and go with, our diets began to change. We began to eat more processed foods, toxins, chemicals and things we normally would not have if we were growing or raising our own food. Many foods marketed "healthy" are in fact just the opposite.

Our grocery stores are filled with products that are marketed to us with promises of them being healthy, nutritious, low fat, gluten free and so much more. Most pre packaged food or ready-made food is actually not good for us. We have been programed to see foods in a certain way, as well as what certain meals should look like.

Breakfast is not in a box

The first myth that we need to discuss is that breakfast is in a box. It does not have to come out of a brightly colored cardboard box with cartoon characters on it. Nor does it have to be poured into a bowl, have milk poured over that and eaten with a spoon.

Breakfast also does not have to be a fluffy circle with a hole cut in it, fried and covered with warm sugar. Nor does it have to be a stack of pancakes, waffles or your classic eggs, bacon and toast.

It is important to start your day with some healthy protein. For some it is easier for them to blend their breakfast of veggies, fruit and protein powder. That is one way to have a quick on the go breakfast that will fire up your body for the day.

Yet leftover chicken or beef with a salad is also breakfast. Hummus and apples can be breakfast. Fresh veggie juice you juice and a hard-boiled egg is another good choice.

Breakfast provides the body and brain with the fuel it needs after running all night. Sleep is the time the body can undergo repair and detoxification. Though we are sleeping our body is working. Even our brains are active while we are sleeping. Muscles and tissues are repaired as we sleep and our hormones are regulated.

When we wake after the sleep period or fast, we need to fuel the body. Hence the word: breakfast! Breakfast gives the body the fuel it needs to start the day and to carry us through the day.

Many studies have shown how eating breakfast can improve memory and concentration levels. Breakfast can also make us happier, it improves our mood and lower stress levels. Studies have shown that when we skip breakfast we make poor food choices later in the day and tend to not only over eat but gain weight.

"According to the Franklin Institute a morning meal high in protein raises your brain's tyrosine levels. This helps your brain produce neurotransmitters called norepinephrine and dopamine, which give you energy and make you feel awake and alert. Protein provides the amino acids your brain needs to function at its optimal level." Maia Appleby

Lunch Not a Sandwich

We grew up taking our lunch to school with us in a lunch box. Most commonly it contained a sandwich, a piece of fruit, a sweet dessert and milk or juice. When we think of lunch we think of sandwiches. Lunch meats between bread with a little lettuce, tomato, onion and maybe cheese. Or perhaps a tuna or chicken salad between bread. We even put Italian meatballs with sauce in bread.

I have had hundreds of people ask me: "What can I eat that is portable if it is not a sandwich?" We are so programed to think that portable food means a sandwich. Even when packing for the beach, a picnic or a bbq, sandwiches are on the list.

"The bread-enclosed convenience food known as the "sandwich" is attributed to John Montagu, fourth Earl of Sandwich (1718-1792), a British statesman and notorious profligate and gambler, who is said to be the inventor of this type of food so that he would not have to leave his gaming table to take supper." Food TimeLine

"Sandwiches first appeared in American cookbooks in 1816. The fillings were no longer limited to cold meat, as recipes called for a variety of things, including cheese, fruit, shellfish, nuts and mushrooms. The years following the Civil War saw an increase in sandwich consumption, and they could be found anywhere from high-class luncheons to the taverns of the working class." Tori Avery

"In the late 1920s, when Gustav Papendick invented a way to slice and package bread, sandwiches found a new audience. Mothers could easily assemble a sandwich without the need to slice their bread, and children could safely make their own lunches without the use of a knife. The portability and ease of sandwiches caught on with families, and the sandwich became a lunchroom staple." Tori Avery

Portable Lunches

There are some decent brands of gluten-free bread on the market now and ways to bake your own gluten free bread. Yet lets look at lunch in a different way. Lets discuss what lunch can look like without it being a sandwich and also how to make some lunch's portable.

Wraps are a great way to make lunch portable. Two very simple ways to wrap food is to use lettuce or cabbage leaves or to use rice paper. Both are portable and you can fill them with all kinds of interesting things from thinly sliced veggies, roasted meats or chicken, salads... the filling ideas are endless.

Rice paper wraps are fun and a light way to take food. They are sold in solid disk shapes, which you dip into a bowl of warm water for a few seconds and then they are pliable. Lay them flat and lay your ingredients in the center and roll up as you would a burrito. I usually put a damp paper towel over the rolls to keep them tender and moist while in transit.

If you want to use cabbage leaves, it is best to blanch them first so that you can make them pliable. I love using both Napa cabbage leaves as well as purple cabbage leaves. Heat a pot of boiling water and drop the leaves in the water for a few minutes. Pull them out and put into a bowl of ice water to shock them. Then dry them and get ready to fill. Once you fill the leaves roll them up like a burrito, tucking in the ends and use a toothpick to keep it closed.

I love butter lettuce wraps so much that it is one of my go to portable food item. I put the leaves in their own container and the stuffing ingredients in another. Then I make them one at a time when it is time for lunch. Romaine lettuce is another good wrap leaf. It is strong enough to be wonderful with burgers. I usually double up the leaves on each side of the burger and tuck the ends around on side of the burger keeping the top part open.

Another great portable lunch item is the salad jar. This is a great way to keep your salad fresh and ready to eat when you are ready. You put the dressing on the bottom of the jar so it does not make the lettuce soggy. You then layer your sturdier ingredients on top of the dressing: garbanzo beans, kidney beans, cherry tomatoes and cucumbers. The last ingredient to go in the jar is the lettuce. When you are ready to eat, give the jar a quick shake to make sure the dressing coats everything!

Skewers of beef, chicken or veggies that have been grilled are great portable lunch ideas. Or things like: chicken or beef satays.

Baked frittatas are a great portable lunch since they can be eaten at room temperature. Fill them with lots of fresh herbs, veggies and some meat. Bake them and cut them into squares. The squares are very portable.

Non-Sandwich Lunches

Salads are great for lunches. Not just the salads made of lettuce but there are so many ways to make salads. Quinoa salads, that you fill full of fresh herbs and veggies. Bean salads where you add roasted onions, cucumbers and fresh herbs. Gluten free pasta salads made with bold flavors. Shredded veggie or fruit salads with chili, lime and exotic seasonings.

Hearty soups make great lunches. The neat thing about soups is that you can put almost anything in them and they turn out delicious. End of the week veggie soup is a great one to clean out your fridge from all the bits of veggies that need to be eaten. Bean soups with or without meat. Roasted vegetable soups, root soups, tomato soups and all kinds of chicken soups. Soups that contain beans, rice, veggies or proteins. The varieties of soups you can make are endless. Soups can even be portable in a thermos.

Similar to soups, stews make a great lunch. Beef stew, chicken stew, lentil stew and roast vegetable stew. Again the options are endless.

Anything you would make for dinner would also make a great lunch. A lot of cultures believe that eating the main meal in the middle of the day is better for your health since it gives you the energy for the rest of the day and you have proper time to digest it.

Professor Carl Johnson, of Vanderbilt University said: "The biological clock controls our metabolism, so the way in which we metabolize the same foods during the day and night is different. If you metabolize food during the day, when you are active, you tend not to convert so much of that to fat. Whereas food eaten during the night or late evening is more likely to be converted into fat."

Take our 8-week companion course and master all of these topics with personal support and help. The course gives you more tools that you can use in your daily life with ease. www.glutensugardairyfree.com/companion-course

What is Healthy Food?

Organic Veggies

"The term "organic" refers to the way agricultural products are grown and processed. Specific requirements must be met and maintained in order for products to be labeled as "organic."

Organic crops must be grown in safe soil, have no modifications, and must remain separate from conventional products. Farmers are not allowed to use synthetic pesticides, bioengineered genes (GMOs), petroleum-based fertilizers, and sewage sludge-based fertilizers." Jeanne Segal, Ph.D.

According to Lawrence Robinson, there is a simple and distinct difference between organic and non-organic.

"Organic produce:
- No Pesticides in production
- Grown with natural fertilizers (manure, compost).
- Weeds are controlled naturally (crop rotation, hand weeding, mulching, and tilling).
- Insects are controlled using natural methods (birds, good insects, traps).

Conventionally grown produce:
- Pesticides used
- Grown with synthetic or chemical fertilizers.
- Weeds are controlled with chemical herbicides.
- Insecticides are used to manage pests and disease."

Much of the fruits and vegetables found in regular markets are not organic. Some of that produces has been genetically modified (GMO's) to make food crops resistant and have a longer shelf life.

Produce that is organic will have an "organic" label on it. You can also find lots of organic food at farmers markets. Organic food not only has fewer pesticides but also is most often fresher. It does not have the chemicals and preservatives that allow for a longer shelf life. Because of that, it tastes better; there is more natural flavor.

According to an article in the Guardian, "Organic food has more of the antioxidant compounds linked to better health than regular food, and lower levels of toxic metals and pesticides, according to the most comprehensive scientific analysis to date.

The international team behind the work suggests that switching to organic fruit and vegetables could give the same benefits as adding one or two portions of the recommended "five a day".

The team, led by Prof Carlo Leifert at Newcastle University, concludes that there are "statistically significant, meaningful" differences, with a range of antioxidants being "substantially higher" – between 19% and 69% – in organic food. It is the first study to demonstrate clear and wide-ranging differences between organic and conventional fruits, vegetables and cereals.

The researchers say the increased levels of antioxidants are equivalent to "one to two of the five portions of fruits and vegetables recommended to be consumed daily and would therefore be significant and meaningful in terms of human nutrition, if information linking these [compounds] to the health benefits associated with increased fruit, vegetable and whole grain consumption is confirmed".

Eating organic is healthier though it can cost a little more. There are some fruits and vegetables that you definitely want organic.

What are GMO's?

"A GMO is an organism whose genome has been altered by the techniques of genetic engineering so that its DNA contains one or more genes not normally found there. Note: A high percentage of food crops, such as corn and soybeans, are genetically modified." Dictionary Reference

"How are Crops Genetically Modified? Foreign DNA is inserted into the primary plant species using one of three methods:

E.coli bacteria is combined with a soil bacteria that causes tumors that allows the foreign bacteria to breach the host plant's cells.
Electricity is applied to the host plant to rupture its cell walls, thus allowing the foreign DNA to invade; or a "gene gun" blasts the engineered DNA directly into the plant's cells.

Because the injected genes can come from bacteria, viruses, insects, animals or even humans, GMOs are also known as "transgenic" organisms. Because genes operate in a complex network in ways that are still not fully understood (as discovered during the Human Genome Research Project), genetic engineering can result in both known and unknown/unintended consequences."
GMO Awareness

GMO's are currently banned in 64 countries around the world.

What GMO's do the Body

Many scientific studies link GMO foods to altered metabolism, liver malfunction, kidney malfunction, inflammation, reduced fertility, food allergies, damage to the heart and damage to the digestive process and they have even been linked to cancer in many studies.

"To date, any studies done that relate to GMOs have been performed on animals, with consistent, documented effects of GMO toxicity, including immune dysregulation (asthma, allergy, and inflammation); accelerated aging; infertility; dysregulation of genes associated with cholesterol synthesis, insulin regulation, cell signaling, and protein formation; as well as altered structure and function in the liver, kidney, pancreas, spleen and gastrointestinal system, stillbirth, birth defects, and early death." GMO Awareness

Organic Master List

- Apples
- Bell Peppers
- Celery
- Cherries
- Cherry Tomatoes
- Cucumbers
- Grapes
- Hot Peppers
- Kale/Collard Greens
- Nectarines
- Pears
- Peaches
- Potatoes
- Raspberries
- Spinach
- Strawberries
- Summer Squash

Non-Organic Master List

Just because they have lower pesticide levels than the vegetables and fruit that need to be organic does not mean they are totally safe for you. These fruits and vegetables have a thicker skin, which protects them from pests, and so less pesticide is used in growing these.

- Asparagus
- Avocado
- Bananas
- Broccoli
- Cabbage
- Cantaloupe
- Cauliflower
- Eggplant
- Grapefruit
- Kiwi
- Mango
- Mushrooms
- Onion
- Papaya
- Pineapple
- Sweet Corn
- Sweet Peas Sweet Potatoes

Antibiotic free meat and poultry

"Organic meat, dairy products, and eggs are produced from animals that are fed organic, non-GMO feed and allowed access to the outdoors. They must be kept in living conditions that accommodate the natural behavior of the animals. Ruminants must have access to pasture. Organic livestock and poultry may not be given antibiotics, hormones, or medications in the absence of illness; however, they may be vaccinated against disease.

Use of parasiticide (a substance used to destroy parasites) is strictly regulated. Livestock diseases and parasites are controlled primarily through preventative measures such as rotational grazing, balanced diet, sanitary housing, and stress reduction." Jeanne Segal, Ph.D.

Conventionally raised meat and dairy are given antibiotics, hormones and are fed with grains that have GMO's in them as well as other animal bi-products in it. A lot of time they are raised indoors and do not have access to the outside, fresh air and growing vegetation.

"Animals raised organically are not allowed to be fed antibiotics, the bovine human growth hormone (rbGH), or other artificial drugs. Animals are also not allowed to eat genetically modified foods. Further, animal products certified as organic cannot have their genes modified (for example, a scorpion gene cannot be spliced into a cow gene).

The animals are raised in a healthier environment, fed organic feed, and often eat a wider range of nutrients than those raised in factory farms (such as would be the case of free-range chickens and ranch cattle). The animals are not from a test tube.

The practice of feeding cattle the ground up remains of their own species may to cause bovine spongiform encephalopathy, a horrific disease that destroys the central nervous system and brain, can be given to humans who eat the cows. The disease in humans has a very long latency period, and is called, Creutzfeldt-Jakob disease

Organically raised animals have been shown to be significantly healthier than their factory-raised counterparts." Annie B. Bond

Some organic meat and poultry have more of omega-3 fats and the reason is their diet. They eat more grass and have lower fat levels than the ones that are fed more grain.

Choosing to eat organic meat and poultry is choosing to know what goes in your body. If you eat conventional meat and poultry and ingest all of the chemicals, it can cause damage to your body and illness.

Fish and Seafood

There are many hidden health dangers in fish and seafood that many are not aware of. Toxic levels of chemicals, bacteria and disease are in some fish and seafood. One of the ways it gets contaminated is the practice of fish farming. Wild caught fish have fewer toxins that farmed fish.

"Many fish-lovers would be horrified to learn that huge quantities of fish and shrimp are now being grown in giant nets, cages, and ponds where antibiotics, hormones and pesticides mingle with disease and waste. These industrialized aquaculture facilities are rapidly replacing natural methods of fishing that have been used to catch fresh, wild seafood for millennia." Food & Water Watch

The fish farmers are actually using genetically engineered fish that grows at twice the normal rate. These are called GE (genetically engineered) animals.

"Ponds enclose fish in a coastal or inland body of fresh or salt water. Shrimp, catfish and tilapia are commonly raised in this manner. Wastewater can be contained and treated. However, the discharge of untreated wastewater from the ponds can pollute the surrounding environment and contaminate groundwater. Moreover, the construction of shrimp ponds in mangrove forests has destroyed more than 3.7 million acres of coastal habitat important to fish, birds and humans." Monterey Bay Aquarium Seafood Watch

"Nearly all fish and shellfish contain traces of mercury. Yet, some fish and shellfish contain higher levels of mercury that may harm an unborn baby or young child's developing nervous system. The risks from mercury in fish and shellfish depend on the amount of fish and shellfish eaten and the levels of mercury in the fish and shellfish." FDA

These fish contain high levels of mercury.

- Shark
- Swordfish
- King Mackerel
- Tilefish

If you are interested in finding out how safe the seafood or fish you want to have is save, you can go to the website called Seafood Watch that is run by the Monterey Bay Aquarium. http://www.seafoodwatch.org/

Take our 8-week companion course and master all of these topics with personal support and help. The course gives you more tools that you can use in your daily life with ease. www.glutensugardairyfree.com/compaion-course

SET UP FOR SUCCESS

My Story

When changing your lifestyle and the way you eat, you have to set yourself up for success. I cringe every January as all of the new fad diets come out, the special gym memberships and New Year Cleanses. If you try to change everything at once, there is a very good chance you will not succeed.

Think of the times you started a new diet or health plan. Perhaps you did very well the first two weeks and then one day you ate things you knew you should not have eaten that were bad for your body. You get discouraged. Then maybe you do it again and tell yourself it is just this one more time. Then you start to feel bad or even gain some weight. It becomes too hard, you tell yourself it does not work. Then you give up and feel bad about it until the next time you try a total overhaul again.

When I started getting healthy I did one thing first. I decided to drink one glass of water more a day. At the time I drank very little water at all. So everyday I made sure to have that glass of water until it became a habit. Soon I was craving water and I no longer had to work at it. I succeeded and then changed another thing and so on. Master one thing first completely and then the next.

When I became gluten, sugar, dairy free for health reasons, I had to set myself up for success. I cleaned out my pantry, freezer and fridge of items I could no longer eat. I took the temptations out of my house. For me that was cream, butter, bread, pasta and sugar treats.

Then I made an inventory of the things I enjoyed eating that was healthy and that were gluten, sugar and dairy free. I was not thinking of replacements for old favorites yet, I was starting basic, just what did I like to eat.

One of my problems was that **I was starving myself fat**. I was not eating enough for my body to have the energy it needed. Because of this, my body stored a lot of fat. So I had to set myself up for success. I had to plan for 3 meals a day and 2 snacks.

It all began by looking at what I did like and not trying to make myself like things that I thought I should like. As soon as I got over the cravings and desire for gluten, sugar and dairy, my taste buds actually changed what they liked. Fruit tasted sweeter than ever. I craved big bold flavors with a lot of different seasonings.

I know if I had begun with forcing myself to eat what I thought I should eat right away, I would have failed. I could not afford to fail since my health was at risk and I wanted to get healthy and have a long life.

I hid my scale. There was no sense in weighing myself every day. It only made me focus on numbers and weight fluctuates every day. I began to notice when my clothes began to feel looser on me. As I began to change my diet and lifestyle my body began to change also. My favorite memory of when I knew the weight was coming off was one day walking from my home office across the living room to the other end of the house and my pants fell down. I was overjoyed to know that my size had changed that dramatically.

I celebrated small success to keep me motivated. I kept and still keep, healthy choices in the house at all times. I plan my meals ahead of time so that I am not caught hungry, tired and overwhelmed. In the beginning I had to really plan since it was a completely new way of eating for me.

I started going to the farmers market every week and talking to the organic farmers. I challenged myself to try at least one new vegetable a week. I would ask how to prepare it and take it home. I began to juice daily and my body began to crave the juice.

Where I use to turn to pre made food, packaged food or fast food, I began to get excited about juice, huge salads, fresh veggies and organic fruit that tasted so sweet. I discovered the variety of nuts and seeds that were good for my body. I made gluten free oatmeal one day with lots of frozen organic berries in it one morning. It was beautiful pink oatmeal that I loved. One morning I tossed chia seeds on top of it as I served it up in a bowl. That oatmeal was one of the best things I had eaten. I would have never thought of doing that in the past.

I began to learn about eating the color of the rainbow, the importance of variety. I started learning about herbs and spices and their benefits on the body. I found combinations of juice that tingled my taste buds and made my body feel good.

Later I began to re-write my cookbooks so that the recipes were all gluten, sugar and dairy free. I discovered flavors I had never tried and became bold in my food choices. What could have been a lack of became a bounty of.

My motivation was how much better I began to feel, how my body began to change, my skin began to look radiant and I looked about 10 years younger. I celebrated (and still do today) every weird dip in my belly as it began to change. The day my cheekbones appeared was a great day! I still am on the journey to health and wellness.

I do not do it with a "have to" mentality but rather a "get to" mentality. I am doing this for me. In the beginning it was a challenge. I developed strategies and ways of making it easier and fun.

Getting Healthy motivation

Take a moment to think about what is motivating you to choose to be gluten, sugar and/or dairy free. Is it food allergies? Is it because you want to be healthier? Is your child allergic and you are learning for them?

Write that Motivation down by hand on paper.

My Motivation:

1. I want to do this because

   _____.

2. I am doing this for

   _____.

3. I will feel better when I

   _____.

4. My goal is

   _____

   ___.

5. If I get discouraged I will

   _____

   ___.

Understanding the triggers

A trigger is: "anything, as an act or event, that serves as a stimulus and initiates or precipitates a reaction or series of reactions." Webster's Dictionary

With food there are three types of triggers: Environmental Triggers, Emotional Triggers and Dietary Triggers.

Environmental Triggers are specific places that you would eat certain ways. It can be a buffet where you might make poor choices, or the movie theater where you get the giant bucket of popcorn, a car trip where you bring foods you don't normally eat and so on. These triggers are brought up in places where you have done the same type of eating for many times. Sometimes we don't even notice we do.

Emotional Triggers are when we turn to food to relieve an uncomfortable emotion. This can be sadness, loneliness, anger or frustration. Instead of dealing with the emotion, you eat to make yourself feel better.

Dietary Triggers are when certain food will cause us to overeat or make bad choices. This can be as simple as taking a whole package of nuts to watch a movie and eating them all. Making a dish of comfort food and eating two servings because it is what you have always done.

With any trigger, it takes you to stop and think about what you are putting in your body, why you are putting it in your body and ask yourself if it is in your best interest before you do. So, if it is an environmental trigger, make a game plan and have a strategy to handle it. If it is emotional, get the support and help you need to relieve the pressure. If it is a dietary trigger, make sure to pay attention to the how and the why of it.

Overcoming Cravings

"In a study from Tufts University, 91% of women said they experienced strong food cravings. And willpower isn't the answer. Feel-good brain chemicals such as dopamine, released when you eat these types of foods, which creates a rush of euphoria that your brain seeks over and over, fuel these urges. What you need is a plan that stops this natural cycle." Prevention

When changing your diet you can unexpectedly be hit by food cravings. I know that when I was giving up gluten, I craved bread for days. So I made sure to eat more veggies from the cabbage family because they kept me full longer. I put purple cabbage ribbons in my salad, steamed up broccoli and sautéed cabbage.

Giving up sugar had me craving sweets and my taste buds had not changed enough to taste the true sweetness of organic fruits. I found that having something sour would drive the craving away. Things like grapefruit, lemon slices, water with lime in it and so on.

The best strategy for overcoming cravings is to have a plan in place. Make sure the foods you crave are on your good list and if they are eat them in moderation. If the foods are on your bad list, have substitutions.

I had a client who was craving potato chips and actually succumbed to the temptation and ate the whole bag. Her body was not happy with that and she got sick for a few days. I suggested exchanging them for lentil chips or hummus chips. Yet only taking a small handful for a serving. She was craving the crunch and the salt.

Sometimes a craving comes along because you are stressed, depressed or sad. It will only make you feel worse to eat something you should not. Find something else to make you feel better and happy. Choose to do something to change your mood instead of feed your mood.

Make sure you are getting enough sleep, drinking enough water and eating enough food to battle cravings. Cravings also occur because you had a habit of doing things in a certain way.

For example when you watch a movie you might have always had popcorn and butter. Plan ahead and make a nice veggie platter (gives you the crunch) and a dairy free dip. Soon you will lose most of the cravings and start reaching for healthy choices.

Baby Steps to Success

Make your goals reachable and realistic. Taking small firm baby steps toward your goal with ensure a positive outcome. Where as giving yourself lofty goals that are hard to attain will give you discouragement.

Celebrate every success so that you can create more success. Every new healthy habit learned is worth acknowledging. From drinking more water, to cleaning out your pantry and filling it with healthy foods to losing those 3 pounds; celebrate.

Build the foundation of your change sturdy. If you were building a house and you rushed your foundation and it was weak and cracked and then built your house on top of that, it would fall over. The wind could just knock it over.
By taking sure baby steps toward your goal, you will build a solid foundation that will have healthy new habits.

Take our 8-week companion course and master all of these topics with personal support and help. The course gives you more tools that you can use in your daily life with ease.
www.glutensugardairyfree.com/compaion-course

Setting up Basic Pantry

Setting up your basic gluten, sugar, dairy free pantry is the key to having the right ingredients on hand when you need them so that you can make meals in minutes. There are some basic items to always have on hand and it will make a big difference if you replenish the items as you use them.

Master Pantry Checklist

Grains

___ Arborio Rice
___ Black Rice
___ Brown Rice
___ Corn Meal/Polenta
___ Gluten Free Oats
___ Organic Masa Harina
___ Quinoa
___ Wild Rice

Nuts & Seeds

____ Brazil Nuts
____ Chia Seeds
____ Flax Seeds
____ Pecan Nuts
____ Pine Nuts
____ Raw Almonds
____ Raw Cashews
____ Walnuts

Legumes

____ Canned Beans
____ Cannellini Beans
____ Dried Beans
____ Garbanzo Beans
____ Kidney Beans
____ Lentils
____ Mung Beans
____ Pinto Beans

Basics

____ Agave
____ Black Pepper
____ Coconut Sugar
____ Corn Starch
____ Curry Paste
____ Himalayan Sea salt
____ Spices
____ Tamari or Coconut Aminos
____ Agave Ketchup
____ Balsamic Vinegar
____ Cocoa Powder
____ Coconut Oil
____ Dijon Mustard
____ Dried Cherries
____ Dried Herbs
____ Dried Raisins
____ Good Olive Oil
____ Good Vinegars
____ Herbal Tea
____ Maple Syrup
____ Medjool Dates
____ Nut Butter
____ Sesame Oil
____ Vanilla

Staples

____ Applesauce Organic

____ Rice Noodles

____ Anchovies

____ Canned Green Chilies

____ Capers

____ Coconut Milk

____ Dried Shitake Mushrooms

____ Fire Roasted Tomatoes

____ Gluten Free Pasta

____ Jar of Marinated Artichoke Hearts

____ Jar of Roasted Peppers

____ Rice Crackers

____ Rice Sheets

____ Stock (chicken, veggie and beef)

____ Tomato Paste

____ Tomato Sauce

____ Tuna

Money Saving Tips - Pantry

The pantry ingredients are important because they are your non perishable ingredients. Things like the organic stock I purchase in bulk at the big box store. I use stock instead of water in rice to make it have more flavor. Things like the fire roasted tomatoes, I stock up on them when they go on sale.

If you are building your pantry from almost scratch, like I did, pick the top five ingredients you would most likely use. Then replenish as you go and once a week when you are doing your normal grocery shopping, pick up another ingredient from the list. Soon you will have a well stocked pantry.

I love to save money when shopping for pantry items. Many times I shop ethnic food stores. I can usually find some of my ingredients much cheaper there. For example, if I need canned or dried beans, the local Mexican Market is the place to go. If I need coconut milk or Thai curry paste, the Asian Market is my choice.

The best practice is to have at least two or three of you most used items like canned tomatoes, coconut milk, types of dried beans, stock and such on hand so that you won't be caught in a pinch. In fact, if you follow the checklist and get the majority of the ingredients, you will be able to make meals just with pantry ingredients should you choose to. Perfect for when you are in a pinch!

Replenishing the pantry items when they are on sale is always the best way to save money! I know that every few months my fire roasted tomatoes go on sale for $10 for 10 cans and I stock up then. I will grab 10-12 cans and know that it will be used at home and that I won't have to purchase them for a while.

At first I set up an extra bookshelf in my garage to handle my pantry overhaul. I have since found a small room that I store all of my things in. Think outside of the box and create a good storage place for the overflow. Shop grocery outlets for pantry items, ethnic markets, big box stores and look at what goes on sale when at your local grocery store.

Setting up Basic Freezer

Setting up your basic gluten, sugar, dairy free freezer is the key to having the right ingredients on hand when you need them so that you can make meals in minutes. There are some basic items to always have on hand and it will make a big difference if you replenish the items as you use them.

Master Freezer Checklist

____ Bacon
____ Berries
____ Chicken Breast Tenders
____ Cooked Rice
____ Cooked Quinoa
____ Fish
____ Frozen Fruit
____ Frozen Veggies (variety)
____ Ginger, Whole
____ Gluten Free Bread
____ Grapes
____ Ground Beef
____ Ground Chicken
____ Herbs
____ Lemon Juice
____ Lemon Zest
____ Ripe Bananas
____ Sausages (chicken, beef or pork)
____ Shrimp
____ Stew Meat
____ Whole Chickens

Money Saving Tips - Freezer

I have some great money saving tips for how to utilize your freezer.

Frozen Cooked Rice
Make cooked rice or quinoa, let it cool and put it in a plastic zip baggie. The plastic baggie means it can lie on a shelf and not take up a lot of room and you can package the rice or quinoa in serving sizes. Then take out the rice or quinoa when you are ready for it and heat it in the microwave or let it defrost on the counter. Great time saver!

Bacon Tricks and Tips
Open your package of bacon. Lay parchment paper on a baking sheet that will fit in your freezer. Place the bacon pieces one at a time on the sheet being careful to not overlap the piece. Freeze. Once frozen drop into a zip baggie. Now when you want to add more flavor to a dish and only need a little bacon, you can pull out individual pieces. This saves on waste and makes the bacon stretch further.

Fresh Herb Tricks

Take fresh herbs like rosemary and chop them up very fine. Put into an ice cube tray and pour melted coconut oil over the herbs or good olive oil. Freeze. Once frozen pop the herb cubes into a baggie. Now when you need them for salad dressing or the base of a sauce, you just drop them in a pan on the stovetop. This can be done with basil, garlic, thyme, sage and parsley.

Lemon Tips

Zest a bag of lemons and freeze the zest in a zip baggie. The zest is great to add to mayo, salad dressings and even to revive pasta sauces. It freezes very well. Juice the juice of those lemons and pour the juice into an ice cube tray and freeze. Once frozen put the cubes in a plastic zip bag. These lemon cubes can be used to add to mayo for a quick lemon aioli, to a sauce for a lemon punch and even added to the stock sauce to make a Chicken Piccata. Lemon juice and zest can add a lot of flavor to dishes. It is even great in salad dressings and marinades.

Ginger

The whole root of ginger freezes very well. It defrosts quickly to dice or slice into rings for use. It even works very well for a punch of flavor for that stir-fry by grating it frozen. Ginger tea helps settle upset stomachs.

Marinades

One of my favorite tricks is to put beef or chicken in a marinade and toss it in the freezer. The day you are ready to cook, simply toss in the fridge in the morning and let it defrost. Or toss it into a bowl of cold water while in the baggie in the marinade to defrost. The neat thing about this tip is as the protein defrosts; the marinade gets into it for tons of flavor. Makes dinnertime easy!

Family Size
Making family size dishes and freezing them in zip baggies in individual servings is another way to stretch the grocery dollars and save time down the road. You can make your own "T.V." dinners by purchasing plastic meal containers and putting the full meal in them: side dish like rice or mashed sweet potatoes, the veggie and the main dish. Then you can pull them out of the freezer when you are ready to eat. This way not only are you saving money and time, but you know what is in your food.

Using it All
Save all of your bones, onion ends, limp carrots, droopy parsley and things that you would normally toss. Put them in a zip bag in the freezer and you can use them to make homemade stock.

Roast a whole chicken and use the carcass to create your own homemade chicken stock you can freeze. You can do the same with veggies or beef bones.

The meat from the whole chicken can be used to create more than one dish. For example you can use the breasts for a beautiful chicken salad and the leg and thigh meat in a red curry with veggies.

Look at how you can use the ingredient in more than one dish to make it go farther.

Sale Savings

Most grocery stores have an area near the butcher that has manager specials. This is where they put the meat and poultry that will expire in a few days but it is still good. This is a great way to save money. When you bring it home, pull it out of the packaging, wrap it in plastic wrap and then put in a plastic zip freezer bag. This way your meat or poultry won't get freezer burn. Do not just toss the package from the store in the freezer, it will get freezer burn.

Setting up Basic Fridge

The setup for the basic fridge is very important for saving money and for making quick easy meals. In the next section of the book you will learn how to prep your food for the week and how to create meal plans.

Master Fridge Checklist

____ Apples
____ Baby spinach
____ Bell peppers
____ Berries
____ Broccoli
____ Capers
____ Carrots
____ Celery cucumber
____ Dijon mustard
____ Eggs
____ Fresh fruit
____ Fresh herbs
____ Fresh veggies
____ Garlic
____ Hummus
____ Lean ground beef
____ Lemons
____ Limes

____ Mayonnaise
____ Mushrooms
____ Nut butter
____ Onions
____ Organic agave ketchup
____ Potatoes
____ Roast chicken
____ Salad
____ Salsa
____ Shredded cabbage
____ Water

Money Saving Tips - Fridge

Farm Direct Deliveries
Ordering fresh organic produce to be delivered from the local farm weekly is a great way to save money on veggies and fruit and to try new ingredients. Most places that do this allow you to adjust what you want in your box each week. That way if you do not like a certain vegetable, you can request that it not be put in and they will make a substitution. Most farms send along information about what is in your box and some recipe ideas also inside of your delivery box.

Making Fresh Herbs Last
If you put your fresh herbs like cilantro and parsley in your crisper drawer, they will only last days and not weeks. If you treat them like flowers, they will last weeks in your fridge. Here is the trick: Trim the ends of the herbs and put them in a glass with a few inches of water and then cover them loosely with a plastic bag. Set the glass on the top shelf of the fridge. Every few days change the water and trim the ends. They will last for weeks this way!

Make a List

Later in this book we will talk about how to make easy meal plans, but the first thing to do is to make a list of what veggies you have in your fridge. This way you will know your options when it comes to meal plans and you will know what you need to use right away!

Cooked Proteins = Quick Meals

Having a whole cooked chicken, some cooked beef and hard-boiled eggs on hand makes mealtime quick. You can always add cooked protein to a salad, a stir fry or put into a nice sauce.

Citrus

Having lemons, limes or oranges on hand is a great trick to adding bold flavor to a salad dressing, marinade or complete meal. Citrus is great for its juice but also for its zest. This is one staple I always have in my fridge.

Garlic

When you are short on time and need garlic it is easier to have peeled garlic. Yet if you purchase peeled garlic at the store it can be expensive and they don't last very long. Here is a quick money saving trick to having peeled garlic on hand. Take a whole head of garlic and drop it into an empty clean jar. Put the lid on the jar. Now shake the jar very hard, the garlic will bang against the bottom and top of the jar as the paper falls off the cloves. When you are done shaking the paper will be on top, the cloves on the bottom. Remove the paper, put the lid back on the jar and place in the fridge until you need garlic cloves.

Take our 8-week companion course and master all of these topics with personal support and help. The course gives you more tools that you can use in your daily life with ease. www.glutensugardairyfree.com/companion-course

Meals in Minutes

This section of the book has all of the tools you need to get healthy, easy and delicious meals on the table in minutes. I will be showing you how to shop and prep for the week ahead. You will learn how to make meals by flavor profile vs recipes (how they taste: Italian, Mexican etc.). I will also show you some conversions and substitutions so you can take conventional recipes and make them gluten, sugar and dairy free! I am including shopping lists that you can use, some simple examples that you can use as base recipes that you can get creative with.

Meal Prep for the Week

Having what you need on hand makes meal prep so much easier. In this section you will learn what to have on hand for the week so that you can make easy delicious meals.

By preparing your veggies and proteins ahead of time, it makes making meals faster. For example if your veggies are blanched ahead of time then the cook time will be far less when doing the meal. Having the meats and chickens cooked ahead of time allows you to quickly drop them in a sauce or a stir-fry to warm through and pick up the flavor from the seasonings of that particular dish.

I normally do my prep for the week on Sundays after I return with my finds from the local organic farmers market. There are some staple vegetables I always get like fresh greens, broccoli and items for salads.

I roast my chickens and beef in the oven or rotisserie as I go to work blanching my veggies and making my salads.

Master Shopping List

PROTEINS

____ Chicken breasts - 4 bone in
____ Ground beef - 2 pounds
____ Hard boiled eggs - dozen
____ Roast beef - 1 small or tri tip
____ Roast chicken - 1 whole
____ Tuna - 2 cans

FRUIT AND VEGGIES

____ Baby spinach
____ Berries
____ Broccoli - 1-pound
____ Bunch green onions
____ Butter lettuce
____ Carrots - 8
____ Chard or kale
____ Cucumbers - 2

____ Fingerling or small potatoes - 1-pound
____ Gluten free oats
____ Head of garlic
____ Lemons - 5
____ Limes - 2
____ Melon
____ Mushrooms
____ Onions - 4
____ Papaya
____ Red bell peppers - 2
____ Salad green mix
____ Shredded purple cabbage
____ Spaghetti squash
____ Sweet potatoes - 3
____ Tomatoes - 6
____ Zucchini - 4

Veggie Prep

Preparing your veggies for the week saves you a lot of time during the week if you do not have to spend your time washing, chopping and cooking them every day. The first thing I do is wash all of my veggies and dry them. The next step is all the chopping. I pull out a large cutting board and get to work.

Bell peppers are seeded and cut into strips. Onions are cut into thin wedges for a stir-fry or curry as well as a few are finely diced for other dishes. Broccoli, squash, mushrooms and carrots are cut into bite size pieces. Garlic is peeled and some is left whole and some is finely diced for dishes later in the week.

I have found that if your veggies are blanched ahead of time, then the cook time will be far less when doing the meal. To blanch a vegetable means that they are dropped in boiling water, which partially cooks them, and then they are dropped into ice water to "shock" them and stop the cooking process. You can also partially steam them and then shock them.

I usually blanch broccoli, green beans, carrots and any other more firm veggies like chayote, parsnips or sugar snap peas. After the veggies are shocked, take them out of the water and spread on dishcloths to dry. You want them to be dry before you package them up for the fridge.

Onions, bell peppers and greens are just prepped but not blanched or steamed. They cook quickly in a stir-fry or sauce.

Slice up your cucumbers and other ingredients also. I use plastic zip baggies for most items because they stack nicely in the crisper drawers and wash them when I empty them so that they can be used again.

The one exception to this is onions and garlic. I either use glass jars or plastic food storage containers for them because it keeps their odor out of the fridge and out of the other food in the fridge.

Salad Prep

The other thing that I make is my salads. I always have a large green salad base made. My favorite one is a mix of baby kale, baby chard, baby spinach and a spring mix. Then I add shredded purple cabbage and shredded carrots to it. I make it in a large bowl and toss it well. Then it is put into large zip bags that can lay one on top of the other in the crisper drawer in the fridge. This takes up less room than a big bowl does.

I always make a lemon quinoa salad with veggies. Sometimes it will have sautéed asparagus and mushrooms, other times it becomes a Tabouli salad with parsley, tomatoes and cucumbers. I cook my quinoa in stock, chicken or vegetable so that it has more flavor. As soon as it is done cooking I toss in the juice of one fresh lemon, stir and cover the pot so the lemon flavor makes the quinoa fluffy and full of lemon flavor. You can put whatever veggies you desire in this to make it your own. The nice thing is that is makes a perfect side dish or meal on its own since quinoa is a source of protein.

I make my lunches also as well as my dinners. I normally have either a chicken salad or a tuna salad made in my fridge for quick meals. I can put a scoop of it on top of the main green salad, sprinkle some aged balsamic vinegar over it, and add some sliced cucumber and tomato, and lunch is made!

I have a variety of chicken salads, sometimes I use apples, celery and madras curry powder (it is a blend of curry powder and other seasonings that I love), other times I might add apple, nuts and grapes. The chicken might be cubed or shredded depending on the type of salad I am making. I shred it if I am making a Thai flavor salad with mint, cilantro and chili or if I am making a Mexican style one with jalapenos, cilantro and cumin. Just pick the flavor you want and add the ingredients to create it!

Tuna salads can have as many varieties. One of my favorites has capers and cilantro in it or dill, celery and a pickle in it. You can add shredded carrots, parsley and lemon to make a tasty salad.

Protein Prep

Having the protein cooked and ready will allow quick meals, as it just needs to heat in a sauce, stir fry or other dish. I also roast my chicken and my beef so that it can be used in salads or in other main dish entrees.

I cube some of the chicken for chicken salads and some I shred that might go in soups or sauces. It is just a personal preference. It saves time when you can grab a handful of cooked chicken and add it to a red curry sauce that is simmering on the stove.

I also brown my ground beef with onions, garlic, salt and pepper and drain the fat off. This means if it is taco night I can add the cooked beef to a skillet, a touch of stock, chili powder and cumin and taco meat is done in just a few moments. Or I can take the beef and add it to some coconut milk, cashew cream, sliced mushrooms, a splash of white wine, black pepper and thyme to create a beef stroganoff. One of my favorites is to take the cooked beef and add coconut milk, fresh basil, salt, pepper and green beans, delicious!

Quick Easy Flavor Profiles

Some of the quickest meals to make don't necessarily need a recipe, rather you need to know what flavor profile you desire. It is the same thing you do when you decide to go out to eat, you choose by flavor profile. You decide you feel like eating Italian tonight or Mexican. Both types of food have very distinct flavors that you recognize right away.

In order for you to make quick meals from the ingredients in your fridge, you need to know some basic flavor profiles. That way that cooked chicken in your fridge or ground beef can turn into a delicious meal!

If you have chicken, ground beef, onion and garlic on hand, it will be easy to turn those four ingredients into many different dishes with flavors from around the world. Same ingredients, different dishes because of the change in the flavor profile.

I am going to cover **5 major flavor profiles**: Italian, Mexican, Middle Eastern, Greek and Asian. Each has specific spices and herbs that make their dishes recognizable. So instead of having to learn and try new exotic ingredients, we will be using what you have in the kitchen right now to take a culinary tour of the world!

Lets begin with Italian flavors. When you think of Italian food you think of sage, basil and oregano. You might think of meatballs in a flavorful tomato sauce with basil and oregano. Chicken with bell peppers, onions, red wine and tomatoes. Chicken with gluten free pasta in a coconut milk and sage sauce. Butternut squash soup with sage. Roasted eggplant with oregano, garlic and onions.

The main spices in Mexican food that are easily recognizable are cumin, chili and cilantro. Lets take the cooked chicken and add chopped tomatoes, onion, garlic, cumin and chili and cook it a bit. Serve it with chopped cilantro. Or take the ground beef and add the cumin and chili to it and make tacos. Add the chicken to stock, with veggies, sliced chilies, lime and fresh cilantro and you have the flavors of Mexico in the bowl of soup.

Three of the main spices in Middle Eastern food are cinnamon, turmeric and cardamom. Strong bold flavors that are easy to recognize. Imagine the chicken with some of the cinnamon and cardamom cooked with onions, garlic, and peppers and served with a turmeric rice. Make beef kabobs with the ground beef and add oregano, cinnamon and cardamom to the beef.

Greek food makes me think of the Greek gyro. The main herbs in Greek food are parsley, oregano and mint. How about a tabbouleh salad made with quinoa, mint, parsley, tomatoes, cucumbers and onions. Even a Greek gyro using a lettuce leaf in place of the pita and putting mini meatballs in the middle that were made with parsley and oregano.

If we were creating Asian style food from the prepped ingredients, we would use ginger, coconut aminos (instead of soy) and lemongrass. Chicken with ginger, garlic, onion, lemon grass, coconut aminos and lime. How about grilling some fresh tuna with orange, ginger and lemongrass for dinner? Ginger beef with mushrooms and a good stock as the base is a nice quick dinner.

Another way to travel through flavor profiles is to purchase a few herb flavor blends or blend them yourself. Some of my favorite to make things quick and easy are:

Chinese 5 Spice Blend: Szechuan peppercorns, cinnamon, fennel seeds, cloves, star anise and salt.

Italian Herb Blend: garlic, rosemary, sage, basil, oregano and thyme.

Taco Seasoning: chili powder, paprika, cumin, oregano, coriander, garlic, salt and pepper.

Take our 8-week companion course and master all of these topics with personal support and help. The course gives you more tools that you can use in your daily life with ease. www.glutensugardairyfree.com/companion-course

Conversions and Substitutions

Substitutions for Items that have gluten:

Flour- use coconut flour, almond flour, amaranth flour

Bread- bread made from tapioca or rice as well as the flours above

Pasta- pasta made from rice, corn, garbanzo beans or quinoa

Soy Sauce- use coconut aminos or tamarind sauce

Substitutions for items that have dairy:

One-cup cow's milk: use one cup of the following: soy milk (plain), rice milk, fruit juice, water, coconut milk or hemp milk.

One-cup of yogurt: use one cup of the following: coconut yogurt, soy sour cream, unsweetened applesauce or fruit puree.

One-stick of butter: use one of the following: 8 tablespoons of coconut oil, 8 tablespoons Vegan Buttery Spread, 8 tablespoons Vegan Organic Shortening, 8 tablespoons vegetable or olive oil or 6 tablespoons unsweetened applesauce + 2 tablespoons on of the others in this list.

Healthy Sugars

Naturally the fiber, vitamins, enzymes as well as the other properties of the fruit or vegetable balance contained sugars in fruit and vegetables.

Some healthy sugars that you might want to consider using are coconut sugar, raw honey and pure maple syrup.

Breads

Commercial Gluten Free Breads, rolls and wraps
Homemade Gluten Free breads, rolls, and wraps
Cauliflower breads, rolls, bagels and pizza crust

Bread Crumbs

Flax Meal
Crushed Nuts
Gluten Free Bread Crumbs
Potato Flakes

Butter

Dairy free margarine like vegan butters

Coconut oil spread

Make your own:

8 tablespoons of coconut oil, 8 tablespoons Vegan Buttery Spread

8 tablespoons Vegan Organic Shortening

8 tablespoons vegetable or olive oil

6 tablespoons unsweetened applesauce + 2 tablespoons on of the others in this list.

Buttermilk

1 Tbsp. of vinegar to 1 cup of milk substitute of your choice

Cheese

Nutritional Yeast

Tofu

Zucchini Cheese

Plant based cheese

Cashew Cream

Cream, condensed and evaporated milks

Coconut milk creamers

Full fat coconut milk

Coconut Cream

Homemade Versions

Eggs

Flax Egg: Begin with whole, raw flax seeds and grind them fresh. One egg equals: 1 tablespoon flax meal plus 3 tablespoons water. Add the ground flax seed to the water and mix well with a fork or mini whisk. Refrigerate for 15 minutes and up to an hour for the egg to set up properly. The ground flax seed forms a sticky goo that is similar to egg whites.

Chia Egg: Using a food processor, spice grinder, or mortar & pestle, grind 1 tablespoon of chia seeds. Soak the ground meal of chia seeds in 3 Tablespoons of warm water for 5 minutes. The seeds will expand and turn into a goopy texture similar to an egg. Chia seeds are gluten-free and grain-free, high in omega-3 fatty acids and are an excellent source of magnesium.

Slurry Binder: For this you can use arrowroot powder, potato or gluten free cornstarch. Mix 2 tablespoons of one of those with 2-3 tablespoons water and mix well before adding to your sauce or other items.

Mashed Fruit Binder: When you are baking something like cookies or sweeter tasting breads you can mash up bananas (1 small) or use ¼ cup of fruit puree. Not only will it give you the moisture of an egg it will naturally sweeten without using any added sugar. A ¼ cup of applesauce works great here too.

Flour Substitutes

Amaranth Flour

Arrowroot Flour

Brown Rice Flour

Buckwheat Flour

Chia Flour

Chickpea Flour

Corn Flour

Cornmeal

Hemp Flour

Lupin Flour

Maize Flour

Millet Flour

Oat Flour-from certified oats

Potato Flour

Potato Starch Flour

Quinoa Flour

Sorghum Flour

Tapioca Flour

Teff Flour

White Rice Flour

Commercial Flour Blends

Homemade Flour Blends

Milk

Almond Milk

Cashew Milk

Coconut Milk Beverages

Coconut Milk

Hemp Milk

Oat Milk

Rice Milk

Pasta

Gluten Free Pasta

Spaghetti Squash

Zucchini Noodles

Sour cream and cream cheese

Commercial substitutes using coconut milk

Plant based cream cheese

Soy Sauce

Coconut Aminos
Gluten Free Soy Sauce
Tamari Sauce

Sugar Substitutes

Stevia
Agave Nectar
Coconut Palm Sugar
Coconut Nectar
Honey
Molasses
Real Maple Syrup
Brown Rice syrup
Rapadura or Sucanat
Yacón Syrup
No Sugar added mashed fruit (for baking)

Yogurt

Coconut milk yogurt

Almond yogurt

Chia Seed Yogurt

      Coconut milk with grass fed gelatin

Whipped Cream

Commercial substitutes

Coconut Cream Whipped

Take our 8-week companion course and master all of these topics with personal support and help. The course gives you more tools that you can use in your daily life with ease. www.glutensugardairyfree.com/companion-course

Part 8: Easy Recipes

Asian Turkey Meatballs

These meatballs pack a bunch of great Asian inspired flavor and are a great meal wrapped in a nice lettuce leaf with some of the dressing drizzled over them. I like to make them mini sized so they fit nicely in the lettuce wraps and they don't dry out during cooking. The trick with ground turkey or ground chicken is to keep the meat moist and add tons of flavor. This recipe does exactly that.

Prep Time: 15 Minutes
Cook Time: 8 Minutes
Yield: 4 servings

Ingredients

Dressing:
2 Tbsp. fish sauce
2 Tbsp. rice vinegar
2 Tsp sesame oil
1/2 Tsp red pepper flakes
1/2 Tsp coconut sugar
Juice of 1 lime

Meatballs:

1 lb. ground turkey

1 Tsp garlic

1 Tbsp. fresh grated ginger

1 Tsp sesame oil

2 Tsp rice vinegar

1 Tsp tamari or coconut aminos sauce

2 Tsp coconut oil for cooking

2 Tbsp. shredded carrots

Instructions:

To make the dressing combine fish sauce, rice vinegar, sesame oil, red pepper flakes, coconut sugar and lime juice in small mixing bowl.

Whisk until incorporated. Set aside.

Prep your garnish by separating the lettuce leaves, rinse and pat dry. Set aside

Dice the cucumber. Set aside

Mince herbs. Set aside

For your meatballs; mince the garlic. Set aside

Grate the ginger. Set aside

In large mixing bowl combine ground turkey, garlic, ginger, sesame oil, rice vinegar and soy sauce.

Stir until just combined, being careful not to over stir and create tough meatballs

Use tablespoon to measure mix and form into balls using your hands.

Heat oil in large skillet on medium heat.

Once the oil is hot, add meatballs.

Brown on all sides, cooking for a total of 5-7mins.

Garnish and serve.

Avocado Chocolate Mousse

One of my favorite desserts after a good meal use to be chocolate mousse. When I went dairy free, I thought the days of having a decadent chocolate thick and rich mousse were over. They were not! In fact, I prefer this avocado mousse to the traditional dairy one. Just note, it will not taste like avocado at all. Use good cacao powder when making this. Once it sets in the fridge, it will be a great sweet chocolate end to a great meal!

Prep Time: 10 minutes
Yield: 4 Servings

Ingredients:

1 ripe avocado
1/3 cup cacao powder
1/4 cup honey
1/4 cup almond or coconut milk
1-2 tsp vanilla extract

Instructions:

Blend all ingredients in blender, scraping down sides until thoroughly mixed.

Chill in refrigerator for 2-3 hours.

Cashew Cream

This is my super secret ingredient that I learned after going dairy free! You will be amazed by what you can do with this cashew cream. You can use it in place of:

* Sour cream
* Ricotta cheese
* Mascarpone

The neat thing about cashew cream is that it is very versatile and when it cooks, it thickens the sauce and adds a richness to it that is even better than dairy cream. The mouth feel of this cream is very important and that is why I recommend using a very high powered blender like a vita-mix when making the cream. You want it as smooth as possible.

The more lemon you add to the cream, the more it tastes like sour cream and the less you add the more it tastes like ricotta or other dairy cream. I love to use this cream in zucchini lasagna, in my chicken divine casserole and so many other ways. Do soak your nuts over night and rinse out the old water before blending.

Prep Time: 5 minutes
Soak Time: 4-6 Hours
Yield: 4 Servings

Ingredients:

1 1/2 cups raw cashews
1/3 cup water
1 teaspoons fresh lemon juice
1/2 teaspoon salt

Instructions:

Soak the cashews in a bowl of water for 4-6 hours or overnight. I prefer overnight. Drain and rinse nuts before using.

In the blender add the cashews, water, lemon juice and salt. Blend until totally smooth.
Use a vitamix blender or other heavy duty one. Food processor works also but you will have to blend longer and continue to scrape the sides.

Cauliflower Fried Rice

When I first heard about cauliflower-fried rice I was skeptical. The idea that cauliflower would taste as good as rice was in intriguing. So I made some.
Wow! Then I tweaked it until I got it just right and that it is easy.

Prep Time: 15 Minutes
Cook Time: 15 Minutes
Yield: 4 Servings

Ingredients:

1 head of cauliflower
1/2 lb. (8 slices) of thick-sliced bacon
2 large eggs
1 Tbsp. minced ginger
3 cloves of garlic, minced
2 carrots diced, about 1 cup
1/2 cup of peas, fresh or frozen
4 green onion, thinly sliced
2-3 Tbsp. tamari
2 Tbsp. coconut oil, divided

Instructions:

Cut the cauliflower into florets, discarding the tough inner core.

Working in batches, pulse the cauliflower in a food processor until it breaks down into rice-sized pieces.

Cook the bacon in a frying pan or in the oven until crispy. Let cook and chop into small bits.

In a medium frying pan, heat 1 tablespoon of the coconut oil.

In a small bowl, scramble the 2 eggs and pour into the skillet. Cook and then chop into small bits.

In a medium frying pan, heat the other tablespoon of coconut oil.

Add the carrots and cook for 2 minutes.

Add the peas and cauliflower rice and mix ingredients well. Lower the heat to medium and cover.

Cook until the cauliflower is done, about 7 minutes.

Uncover and stir in the bacon, eggs, green onions, and tamari and serve.

Cauliflower Pizza Crust

Cauliflower is being made in "rice", "bread" and even "pizza crust" these days. It is actually very easy to do and a great gluten free version with all the goodness of a veggie.

I was at a vegan restaurant with a friend and they had a vegan "cheese" pizza on the menu. I had to try it. It was made with a cauliflower crust, vegan cheese, thin slices of tomato and basil.

Prep Time: 10 Minutes
Cook Time: 30 Minutes
Yield: 1 Crust

Ingredients:

1 head cauliflower
2 Tbsp. coconut oil divided
1 egg
1/2 Tsp salt
1/4 Tsp black pepper
1/2 cup vegan cheese (cheddar or mozzarella)

Instructions:

Preheat oven to 450°

Line a cookie sheet with parchment paper and rub 1 Table coconut oil all over it

Cut the cauliflower into florets, removing the core.

In batches in a food processor with a grating blade, grate the cauliflower. (This can also be done with a hand grater.)

Heat a large frying pan with the remaining coconut oil. Add the cauliflower rice to the pan. Cook over medium-low heat for 15 minutes, stirring occasionally. The cauliflower will be soft when done.

In a large bowl beat the egg well.
Add the cauliflower rice, salt, pepper and vegan cheese. Mix well.

Shape mixture in a large circle on the parchment paper

Bake for 13-15 minutes, until golden brown.

Chicken Divan Casserole

This recipe is my version of the classic chicken divan that was so popular in the 1960's and 1970's. The original dish was made with cream of chicken soup, mayo, sour cream and cheddar cheese. I replaced all of those ingredients with cashew cream and coconut milk. Then I added more flavor with lemon juice, madras curry powder and good white wine. The cashew cream thickens the sauce as it bakes in the oven. The result is a very tasty dish that is similar to the original but dairy free and much more healthy.

Prep Time: 20 Minutes
Cook Time: 60 Minutes
Yield: 4 Servings

Ingredients:

2 large roasted chicken breasts
4 cups broccoli florets
1/2 coconut milk
1/2 cup cashew cream
Zest one lemon
Juice of one lemon
1/4 white wine
1/4 teaspoon black pepper
1/2 teaspoon salt
2 teaspoons madras curry powder
Sprinkle of salt and pepper

Instructions:

Preheat oven to 350°

Steam the broccoli until it is just fork tender. Put on a platter. Sprinkle with salt and pepper. Let cool.

Dice the chicken breasts into cubes.

In a large bowl mix the coconut milk, cashew cream, lemon zest, lemon juice, white wine, black pepper, sea salt and madras curry powder.

Add the cooled broccoli and cubed chicken to the sauce. Stir gently until everything is coated in the sauce.

Pour into a small baking dish using your spatula to flatten out the top of the casserole.

Cover tightly with foil.

Bake for 30 minutes covered and another 30 minutes uncovered.

Let sit for 5 minutes so that the sauce can settle. Enjoy!

Classic Green Juice

I love to start my day with a big glass of green juice. It not only gives me energy but it has helped me with my weight loss. When I don't juice for a few days I notice a big difference.

One of the reasons that people don't juice is because there are so many ingredients and it is a big process to get out each one, juice and then clean the juicer. I have found a way around that. The first step is to purchase your ingredients and wash them. The next step is to make individual bags with all the ingredients for green juice in each bag.

Now when it is time to make green juice you just grab a pre-made juice bag. I have timed the process. It takes 5 minutes exactly to juice the bag, wash the juicer and pour your juice! Since I started doing this process, I don't skip juice days as often.

Each bag makes about 3-4 cups of juice. I like to drink a large amount in the morning. Feel free to divide this recipe in half and make smaller juice bags for yourself. I use all organic ingredients. Some people add lemon juice to this recipe.

The green juice should be drunk at once. It loses its nutrients quickly. I do not suggest making a pitcher and keeping it in the fridge. If you want to keep it, blend it with a little coconut water instead of juicing. This process allows the nutrients to stay longer and you can make it ahead of time. Personally, I prefer to juice it.

I noticed this past winter I did not catch colds, the flu or my normal sinus infections. Is it the juice? I believe that the juice played a big part in keeping me healthy.

Yield: 1 Serving

Ingredients:

1 green apple
1/2 English cucumber
1/2 head of celery (using all of it)
1/2 bunch curly parsley
2 inch piece of ginger root
2 big handfuls of kale (I use baby kale)
2 big handfuls of spinach (I use baby spinach)
3 oz. aloe juice

Instructions:

Place first 7 ingredients in a blender or juicer and blend until smooth. Place aloe juice in bottom of glass and pour green juice over.

Classic Pot Roast

Some of my favorite memories of the winter include the smell of a pot roast cooking slowly in the oven. The aromas of the onions, garlic, wine and beef fill the air. I wanted to create a recipe that would work for two people since most pot roast recipes are for the whole family. Pot roast is such a classic comfort meal.

If you do want to make a family size pot roast use a 3-4 pound chuck roast and triple all the rest of the ingredients. Either small or large, this is one delicious meal!

Prep Time: 10 Minutes
Cook Time: 2 Hours
Yield: 2-3 Servings

Ingredients:

1 lb. chuck roast
1 small yellow onion chopped
1-cup red wine
1/2-teaspoon salt
1/2-teaspoon dried oregano
2 tablespoons coconut oil
1/2 of a 15 ounce can fire roasted diced tomatoes
3 small carrots chunked (or 2 large ones)

2-3 red potatoes quartered
3 cloves of garlic minced
1 cup beef stock
1/4-teaspoon pepper
1 bay leaf

Instructions:

Season meat with salt and pepper on both sides.

Sear both sides of the roast in coconut oil in a Dutch oven until brown.

Add wine, stock, garlic, tomatoes, salt, pepper, oregano, bay leaf and onion to pan.

Bring to boil.

Put in 350° oven.

Bake covered 1 hour 45 minutes.

Add potatoes and carrots to pan, stir. (Add more stock if needed to cover the ingredients)

Bake 45 minutes more.

Taste to see if you need to add more salt or pepper.

Serving suggestions: Second serving freezes well. The second half of the diced tomatoes can be frozen for another time. Use good red wine in sauce because the flavor intensifies as it cooks down.

Coconut Chia Seed Pudding

I discovered that chia seeds were really good for me. So at first I started sprinkling them on my daily oatmeal. I loved the crunch in the oats. Then I started thinking that a dessert would be a good idea. I looked in the pantry and found coconut milk and the rest is history. Chia pudding was discovered and devoured.

Prep Time: 5 Minutes
Yield: 2 Servings

Ingredients:

1 can organic coconut milk
1 tsp pure vanilla extract
1/4 tsp sea salt
1/4-cup chia seeds
1/4-cup shredded unsweetened coconut
1/2-cup fresh raspberries or mixed berries

Instructions:

In a pitcher add coconut, chia seeds, coconut milk, vanilla and salt

Mix until very well combined.

Place in the refrigerator and allow to chill for at least 2 hours

Serve with fresh raspberries, mixed berries or a fruit of your choice.

Cold Sesame Cucumber Noodles

I use to love spicy peanut noodles. They were cold pasta noodles that had been tossed into a spicy peanut butter sauce. This is my version of it made with cucumbers instead of wheat pasta and the use of the healthier sunflower seed butter instead of peanut butter. Best to make a double batch, these are addictive! They are great by the bowl full or as a tasty side dish for some grilled chicken.

Prep Time: 20 Minutes
Cook Time: 20 Minutes
Yield: 4 Servings

Ingredients:

1 tsp sesame seeds
2 English cucumbers
1 Tbsp. tahini
1 Tbsp. organic sunflower seed butter (almond will work also)
1 tsp sesame oil
1 Tbsp. coconut aminos (or soy sauce)
1 Tbsp. rice wine vinegar
1 Tbsp. water
1/2 tsp red pepper flakes
2 cloves garlic, crushed
1/4 tsp powdered ginger
1 green onion thinly sliced

Instructions:

Preheat oven to 325°

Spread sesame seeds on baking sheet in even layer and bake until seeds are fragrant and light golden brown.

Peel cucumber and turn into noodles using julienne slicer.
Whisk the remaining ingredients in a medium bowl.

Pour sauce over noodles and mix to coat all the noodles.

Sprinkle toasted sesame seeds over the top and serve.

Eggs in Potato Basket

This is a super easy breakfast or brunch dish that looks so fancy it is perfect to serve guests for holidays. Personally I love when the oven can do the work for me and I get the rewards. So I make this for myself.

In this recipe, I have you shred your own potatoes because it is easy, but if you are in a rush, you can use a bag of those freshly grated potatoes you find at the store. They will do in a pinch.

I like to cook my eggs until the whites set up, but the yolk is runny. This way the potato basket can soak up the yolk when I cut into it.

Prep Time: 5 Minutes
Cook Time: 55 Minutes
Yield: 6 Servings

Ingredients:

3 Russet Potatoes
6 fresh eggs
1/2 teaspoon salt
1/4 to 1/2 teaspoon black pepper
3 tablespoons coconut oil divided

Instructions:

Preheat oven 350°

Peel and grate the potatoes. You can use a hand grater or the food processor.

Take the grated potatoes and put into a cheesecloth or kitchen towel, squeeze all the water out of them.

Put in a bowl and toss with the salt, pepper and 2 tablespoons of melted coconut oil. Mix well using your fingers.

Take the 1 tablespoon of coconut oil and grease the insides of 6 muffin tins.

Put the shredded potato mixture evenly in the six greased muffin tins. Use your fingers to press down on the sides and bottoms of the potatoes to make a nest.
Bake in oven 35-40 minutes until brown. Remove tray from oven leaving nests in the muffin tin to cool. (You can do this step a few hours ahead of time.)

Gently crack one egg in each nest.

Put tray in oven and cook until desired doneness 8 – 12 minutes.

Remove the nests from the muffin tin and serve.

Fennel Kale Soup

The fennel is such a nice addition to this kale and white bean soup. This is an easy soup to make with a lot of flavor that is good enough to serve to company. I made it one day when I was cleaning out the fridge and my plan was to use up the veggies in a soup. I had forgotten that I had picked up fennel at the local farmers market so I added it to the soup along with some ground fennel seeds to boost the flavor. The fresh lemon juice at the end allows the flavors to explode.

.

Prep Time: 15 Minutes
Cook Time: 45 Minutes
Yield: 6 Servings

Ingredients:

2 Tbsp. coconut oil
1 1/2 cup onions
2 cloves garlic
2 tsp salt
2 tsp ground fennel seeds
2 cup diced fennel
1 cup diced carrots
1 1/2 cup diced potatoes
2 tsp thyme
1/4 tsp black pepper

1-15 oz. can fire roasted tomatoes
3 cups cooked white beans
4 cups vegetable or chicken stock
5 cups kale
Juice of one lemon

Instructions:

Dice the onion, mince the garlic and chop the kale.

Dice the fennel, carrots and potatoes in evenly sized small pieces.

In large soup pot, heat the oil over medium heat.

Sauté the onions, garlic, salt, fennel, carrots and potatoes until veggies are fork tender.

Add the fire roasted tomatoes, stock, ground fennel seeds, thyme and black pepper to the veggies. Stir to combine.

Bring to a simmer and cover. Cook for 30 minutes.

Add the drained beans and chopped kale to the soup and stir. Simmer for another 15 minutes.

Mix in lemon juice just before serving.

Garlic Shrimp

I love shrimp and garlic together. One day I realized it was after two in the afternoon and I had not eaten. I needed a quick tasty lunch. I always have frozen raw shrimp in the freezer. They defrost under running water in minutes. This is such a simple dish with simple clear flavors. I found that there are many ways to serve the shrimp once cooked. Some simple ways are over a spinach salad, with side dishes or tossed with noodles and olive oil. This is a perfect recipe for a quick healthy meal.

Prep Time: 10 Minutes
Cook Time: 5 Minutes
Yield: 4 Servings

Ingredients:

24 large shrimp (21/25 count)
4-5 minced cloves of garlic minced
3 tablespoons coconut oil
1/4 teaspoon red chili flakes

Instructions:

Peel and devein the shrimp.

Rinse and dry well.

Heat coconut oil in a large skillet over medium low heat.

Add the garlic and pepper flakes.

Cook for one minute.

Add the shrimp.

Cook for 4 minutes or until done turning once. The shrimp will begin to turn orange and curl into a "C" shape when done. Do not overcook.

Serving Suggestions: Good over a spinach salad. Serve with rice and a vegetable. Chill and eat cold or put over a salad when cold. Can use more pepper flakes for more spice. Toss with gluten free pasta noodles and a little of the noodle water and olive oil to create a sauce.

Gourmet Chicken Stroganoff

My happy place is in recipe creation, food flavor profiles and in the kitchen. So after a stressful day, I had a craving for a big bowl of beef stroganoff. I decided to indulge my desire and create a gluten dairy free version that would still taste delicious, be comforting and enjoyable. When I went to the kitchen to create my new dish, I only had chicken on hand. So my gourmet chicken stroganoff was created.

Prep Time: 10 Minutes
Cook Time: 35 Minutes
Yield: 4 Servings

Ingredients:

3 tablespoons coconut oil divided
1 small yellow onion or half of a normal one diced
1-2 diced cloves of garlic
4-5 fresh shiitake mushrooms sliced
1/3 cup of diced chanterelle mushrooms
1/2 cup good white wine
1/2 cup good chicken stock
1 1/4 cup coconut milk
1/2 teaspoon thyme
1/2 teaspoon salt
1/4 teaspoon fresh ground black pepper

1 large boneless skinless chicken breast or 2 normal size ones sliced
1 package gluten free pasta cooked

Instructions:

Heat 2 tablespoons of coconut oil in a large skillet on medium heat. Add the diced onions and garlic and sauté until translucent.

Add the sliced and diced mushrooms and cook until mushrooms are tender. Cook for about 3 minutes.

Add the white wine and cook 2-3 minutes until the wine is almost completely evaporated.

Add the stock, coconut milk, thyme, salt and pepper.

In another small frying pan, add the coconut oil and cook over medium heat the strips of chicken breast until done. This takes about 2 minutes a side.

Add the cooked chicken to the sauce. Bring up to a boil and then lower to simmer for 10 minutes stirring occasionally. The sauce will thicken naturally

Add the cooked pasta to the sauce and mix well. Let cook together for 2 minutes so that the noodles soak up the flavorful sauce.

Guatemalan Black Beans

A few years ago I went to Panajachel, Guatemala with my best friend. It is located on Lake Atilan, which is surrounded by three volcanos. It is beautiful and I had spent part of my childhood there. One of the staples that we were fed every morning were black beans. These were not your ordinary black beans. These black beans had a lot of flavor but were pureed and thick enough to eat with a fork.

In this recipe, I used a pressure cooker to cook the beans because it infuses the flavor into them directly. This recipe can be adapted for stove top, in that case you will have to cook them for an hour and a half.

A few bean making tips:

Pick through beans before soaking for small pebbles.
Always soak overnight in a large bowl with cool water.
Do not cook beans in soaking water, rinse first and use fresh water.
Never add salt until they are cooked and at the very end.

Prep Time: 8 Hours
Cook Time: 20 Minutes
Yield: 8-10 Servings

Ingredients:

1 1-pound bag of black beans
1 32-ounce carton of good vegetable stock
1 small yellow onion
3 large whole garlic cloves peeled
1 bay leaf
2 tablespoons cumin and 1 tablespoon reserved
2 tablespoons Ancho chili powder and 1 tablespoon reserved
1 tablespoon oil (I used coconut oil)
1 teaspoon salt (or to taste) added at the end only

Instructions:

Soak the black beans overnight, changing the water once.

When you are ready to cook, rinse the beans under cool water.

Chop the onion into large chunks and peel the garlic cloves.

In the pressure cooker, put all the ingredients except the salt and close the lid.

Bring up to 15psi pressure and cook for 20 minutes using the natural steam release method. (If you are cooking on the stove top, bring up to boil and then lower to simmer with lid part way on. Cook for about an hour. Check for doneness.)

Cool and drain the beans keeping the liquid in a separate bowl.

Remove the bay leaf.

Put beans in food processor or blender.

Add salt and some of the liquid.

Blend, adding liquid until you get your desired consistency.

Taste for seasonings. (I added 1 tablespoon each of cumin and Ancho chili powder more to the beans.)

You can also eat the beans without blending. They are delicious whole just like that, just add salt and taste for seasonings. You could also add a jalapeño chili pepper to the beans while cooking for heat.

If cooking stove-top, cook for about an hour and a half.

Hemp Seed Pesto

Wanting to create a new pesto recipe and having learned about how much protein and nutrients are in hemp seeds, I thought I would experiment with using hemp seeds in pesto. After a few tries I found the perfect combination of ingredients and did not even miss the parmesan cheese like I thought I would. This easy pesto lasts up to a week in the fridge in a sealed jar.

Prep Time: 5 Minutes
Yield: 8 Servings

Ingredients:

1 cup Basil leaves, washed and spun dry
1/4 cup Extra Virgin Olive Oil
1 clove garlic minced
1/2 cup Hulled Hemp Seed

Instructions:

Combine basil, garlic, and olive oil in a blender or food processor and blend until smooth.

Add hemp seed and blend just until mixed well. Serve immediately or store in a covered container for up to a week.

Lemon Asparagus Noodles

I bought some beautiful asparagus and peas at the farmers market. It was a warm summer's night and I wanted something fresh for dinner. So I made a gluten free pasta with the veggies, garlic, and lemon. White wine, basil and mint. It was delicious! I ate the leftovers cold the next morning and it was still good!

Prep Time: 10 Minutes
Cook Time: 15 minutes
Yield: 2 Servings

Ingredients:

1 tablespoon coconut oil
2 cups of asparagus cut into one inch pieces
1/2 cup shelled peas
3-4 cloves of garlic minced
1/4 yellow onion finely minced
1 cup good white wine
1 cup vegetable stock
Zest of a whole lemon
Juice of a whole lemon
1/4 cup mint leaves
1/4 cup basil leaves
1/2 teaspoon salt
1/2 teaspoon black pepper
1/2 pound any style gluten free noodles

Instructions:

Put a large pot of water on the stove to boil to cook the noodles.

Add the peas and asparagus to the boiling water and cook for two minutes.

Drain and put into a bowl that has ice and water in it to shock the veggies and stop them from cooking. Drain.

Dice the onion very fine.

Mince the garlic. I used 4 giant cloves because I wanted it to have a lot of garlic. I do all the prep ahead of time. That way cooking the meal is easier and neater!

Heat a large skillet and add the coconut oil.

Once it is hot, add the garlic and onions.

Cook until the onions are translucent and do not let the garlic brown.

Add the white wine and let it reduce over medium heat 3-4 minutes.

Add the vegetable stock, lemon zest, juice of the lemon, salt and pepper to the pan and reduce about 5 minutes. Taste for seasoning.

Cook the pasta, drain it and immediately add to the sauce. Add 1/4 cup of the water from the pasta to the sauce. Toss the noodles well. Add the veggies and the herbs and toss well. Let pasta sit in pan for about 3 minutes covered so that the pasta absorbs the sauce and flavor.

Lemony Quinoa Tabouli

This is one of my favorite salads! I love Tabouli, but I don't eat the bugler wheat it is normally made with any more, so I developed this recipe using quinoa. This recipe has all the flavor profile of the original plus extra lemon and it turns out delicious! I like a lot of flavor in my Tabouli, so use the freshest ingredients you can for the best results.

Prep Time: 20 Minutes
Cook Time: 15 Minutes
Yield: 1 Serving

Ingredients:

1/3 cup good organic virgin olive oil
1/3 cup fresh squeezed lemon juice
1 clove of garlic minced
1/2 cup packed mint leaves
1/2 teaspoon fresh ground black pepper
3/4 teaspoon salt
3 green onions
1 bunch parsley
3 large roma tomatoes or 4 small ones
1/2 English cucumber
1 cup uncooked quinoa

Instructions:

First make the dressing by combining the olive oil, lemon juice, garlic, mint, salt and pepper in a blender.

Pour into a large mixing bowl and set aside.

Cook the quinoa according to package directions. It is usually 1 cup quinoa to 2 cups of water.

Bring to a boil, cover and simmer 10-15 minutes.

As soon it is done, immediately put the hot quinoa into the dressing and mix well. This way the quinoa will soak up all of the flavor. Set aside to cool.

Finely chop the parsley and the green onions and put into a bowl.

Cut the cucumber and take out the seeds. Chop and add to the bowl.

Seed the tomatoes, dice and add to the bowl. Stir together gently.

Add this mixture to the cooled quinoa mixture and toss gently.

Cover and refrigerate for at least an hour so the flavors come together. I like to make this a day ahead.

Lentil Soup

This is an easy to make hearty soup. I love lentils and they come in many colors. I think I used green ones when I wrote this recipe. In doing some research, I even found heirloom brands of lentils. This is a pretty classic recipe with carrots, onions, celery and fire roasted tomatoes. It is one of my go to recipes that always turns out delicious.

Prep Time: 20 Minutes
Cook Time: 45 Minutes
Yield: 6 Servings

Ingredients:

2 cups dried lentils (green or red)
32 ounce box of vegetable or chicken broth
4 carrots peeled and diced
2 celery stalks diced
1 yellow onion diced
3 cloves of garlic minced
1 can fire roasted tomatoes
2 tablespoons tomato paste
1 tablespoon coconut oil
1 teaspoon dried thyme
1/2 teaspoon dried oregano
1/2 teaspoon cumin
1 teaspoon salt
Fresh black pepper

Instructions:

In a soup pot heat the coconut oil over medium heat.

Add the onions, garlic, carrots and celery

Cook until onions are translucent, about 6-7 minutes.

Add the lentils, tomatoes, broth and all the seasonings.

Stir to combine.

Bring up to a boil and then lower the heat to simmer and cover.

Cook 35-40 minutes until the lentils are tender.

Or

After the vegetables have cooked, place them and all the rest of the ingredients into a slow cooker and cook low 8-10 hours or on high for 4-5 hours.

Maple Dijon Chicken

I wanted to create a chicken dish that was a little different, easy to do and came out perfect every time. I started thinking of flavors and came across my pure maple syrup that my friend from Canada had brought me. The dish turned out perfectly and it has become one of my more popular dishes with my readers.

Prep Time: 15 Minutes
Cook Time: 60 Minutes
Yield: 4 Servings

Ingredients:

4 bone in skinless chicken breast
1/4 cup Dijon mustard
3 tablespoons pure maple syrup
1 tablespoons coconut oil
Pinch of red pepper flakes
1/2 teaspoon pepper
1/2 teaspoon salt
Zest of 1/2 lime
2 tablespoons + extra for garnish chopped parsley
1 large clove of garlic

Instructions:

Combine Dijon mustard, garlic clove, parsley, maple syrup, red pepper flakes, salt, black pepper and lime zest into a blender and blend well, scraping sides periodically until it is all incorporated.

Remove 2 tablespoons of the mixture and save for later in a small bowl.

Pour the remaining marinade into large plastic zip bag and add the chicken breasts. Marinate in the refrigerator overnight, at least for a minimum of four hours for best results.

Preheat oven to 350° degrees Fahrenheit.

Rub the inside of a large baking dish with the oil.

Pour the contents of the zip bag into a large baking dish and arrange the chicken breasts bone side down. Bake for one hour.

Use reserved 2 tablespoons of marinade to baste chicken during the last 15 minutes.

Remove from oven, pour any extra sauce over the breasts and garnish with a little chopped parsley.

Morning Detox Tea

Drinking this lemon tea first thing in the morning is great for your body. It wakes up the liver to flush the toxins out of your body; it gives you energy and resets the metabolism.

Yield: 1 Serving

Ingredients:

8 Oz. of hot water
Juice of 1 Lemon
1 teaspoon. Cinnamon
1 tablespoon local raw organic honey

Instructions:

Put the ingredients in a mug and mix well with a spoon.

Ranch Dressing

I wanted a dairy free ranch dressing to go with a Cobb salad I had made. I knew that traditional ranch dressing had dairy. My final version tastes so good and you would not know it has coconut milk in it because of all of the fresh dill, and it tastes like traditional ranch dressing! This dressing also works great as a dip for veggies.

Prep Time: 15 Minutes
Yield: 2 cups

Ingredients:

1 cup mayo
1 1/4 cup coconut milk
3 tablespoons fresh chopped dill
3 cloves of garlic made into a paste with sea salt (use the flat side of your knife to do this)
1 1/2 teaspoons apple cider vinegar
3/4 teaspoon black pepper
1/8 teaspoon salt

Instructions:

Put all the ingredients into a blender and blend until smooth. (I actually put all the ingredients into a large glass jar and shake well.)

Roasted Pork Chops

This is a nice, easy to make, hearty dish. The pork cooks perfectly and all of the flavors of the veggies and seasonings make you want to have second helpings!

Serves: 4
Prep Time: 15
Cook Time: 60 minutes

1/2 teaspoon dried oregano leaves
1/2 teaspoon dried thyme leaves
1/2 teaspoon salt
1/2 teaspoon coarse ground pepper
4 pork rib chops, 1/2 inch thick (1 pound)
1 small bag of red potatoes, about 3 cups quartered
3-4 carrots peeled and cut into 1 inch pieces
1 med yellow bell pepper cut into strips
2 medium onions cut into thin wedges
2 red tomatoes cut into wedges
1 head garlic peeled
2 tablespoons melted coconut oil

Instructions:

Pre heat oven to 400° Fahrenheit

In a large bowl mix the carrots, potatoes, bell pepper, onions, tomatoes and garlic. Add the coconut oil, salt, pepper, thyme and oregano and mix well.

Season the chops with salt and pepper on both sides.

Pour the veggie mix into the bottom of a baking dish. Lay the pork chops on top of the mixture.

Bake uncovered on the middle rack in the oven for 45 minutes.

Take the dish out of the oven, put the chops on a plate and mix the veggies. Then put the chops back on top of the veggies, the other side up.

Bake for another 15-20 minutes until the meat is at 145 degrees Fahrenheit.

Pull the dish. Put the chops on a plate to rest for 3-5 minutes.

Stir the veggies before serving.

Sautéed Spinach

I took myself to dinner to a steakhouse when I was out of town on business. I ordered a steak and a side of sautéed spinach. I could not get enough of the sautéed spinach because it was the best I have ever had. The waiter asked the chef for the recipe but he would not give it up. The chef did send me two more side dishes of spinach on the house since I made such a big deal about it. I ate it all and took my steak home!

I have been on a mission to recreate this spinach dish. I have tried all kinds of ways. I did it and even better! Now I am addicted to this dish! In fact I just ran to the grocery to pick up another 2 bunches of spinach!

Remember that when cooking spinach it really shrinks down, so you will need more than you think you do. Always wash your spinach. The water in my sink is always so dirty after I wash spinach. There is always some dirt mixed in with the leaves.

Prep Time: 20 Minutes
    Cook Time: 5 Minutes
    Yield: 2-3 Servings

Ingredients:

1 bunch of fresh spinach, washed, dried and the stalks pulled off
1 tablespoon organic extra virgin coconut oil
2 cloves of garlic
Sea salt
Fresh ground black pepper
1 tablespoon rice wine vinegar

Instructions:

Chop the cloves of garlic very fine.

Then sprinkle with a little sea salt.

Using the back of your knife (the flat side) press and scrape across your cutting board the garlic.

Do this until the cloves make a paste.

Heat the oil with the garlic and the black pepper. I like flavoring the oil before the spinach goes in because that way the spinach picks up all the flavor.

Once the oil is hot, add your spinach leaves.

Toss with tongs making sure all the leaves get some of the flavored oil.

Near the end, when they are almost all totally wilted, add the vinegar. You usually have 15-30 seconds left of cooking at this point because spinach cooks so fast. This dash of vinegar is what makes this dish come alive!

You can also add a chopped clove of garlic to the olive oil mixture if you want chunks of garlic also. The paste is important because it then coats all of the leaves.

Slow Cooker Pepper Steak

Some days I feel lazy, want my house to smell like good food cooking and have an easy delicious dinner at the end of the day. This recipe is one of those easy, go to recipes that always work out and is delicious. I have even served it to company and they raved. Put this one in your list of quick, easy and tasty go to recipes.

Prep Time: 15 Minutes
Cook Time: 3-4 hours on high and 6-8 hours on low
Yield: 6-8 Servings

Ingredients:

2 pounds sirloin
2-3 cloves garlic
2 sliced bell peppers
1 can stewed tomatoes
1/2 cup beef stock
1 tablespoons corn starch
2 tablespoons fresh grated ginger (2 teaspoons dried)
1/2 teaspoon salt
1/2 teaspoon pepper
1 tablespoons chopped cilantro
2 or 3 lime slices

Instructions:

Slice sirloin into strips, slicing across the grain into one inch strips.

Heat a large frying pan on medium high heat.

Once pan is hot set sirloin strips in and let sit 2-4 minutes or until they release from pan easily. You don't need oil since the natural liquid from the beef will release into the pan.

Flip and brown other side. Remove sirloin from heat on to platter.

Whisk stock with cornstarch and add to slow cooker. If you don't have beef stock, chicken or vegetable stock will work just fine. Use stock, never water!

Add all other ingredients (except cilantro and lime) to slow cooker and stir to combine.

Add sirloin to slow cooker and gently mix well. Cover.

Set on high and cook for 3-4 hours or low for 6-8 hours. Stir once during the cooking. Chop cilantro and cut lime slices and set aside.

Once the beef has cooked, taste and check to see if you need to add more salt or pepper before serving. Many times you do.

I usually serve this dish over brown rice. I put the brown rice on plate and the meat mixture over, topping it with cilantro and a squeeze of lime.

Stuffed Poblano Pepper

I love stuffing peppers of all types. This poblano pepper is a little bit spicy so it naturally needed to be stuffed with Mexican flavors. If you want a really soft pepper, blanch it before stuffing and baking. I like a little bit of texture to my pepper so I just stuff it and bake it. If you cannot find a poblano pepper, which looks like a fat green chili, bell peppers work well also.

Prep Time: 20 Minutes
Cook Time: 35 Minutes
Yield: 1 Serving

Ingredients:

1 poblano pepper
2 tablespoons onion
1 roma tomato
1 garlic clove
1/2 cup black beans
1-teaspoon coconut oil
1/4 teaspoon chili powder
1/4 teaspoon cumin
1/2 cup Yukon gold potatoes (1 medium potato)
1/2 cup and 2 tablespoons vegan pepper jack cheese
1/8 – 1/4 teaspoon salt

Instructions:

Seed and chop the tomato.

Dice the onion and the potato. Rinse the beans.

Sauté the onion, garlic, and potato in the coconut oil over medium heat.

Cook 5 minutes. The potatoes will be tender and the onions translucent.

In a bowl, add the sauté mixture, black beans, tomato, chili powder and cumin. Mix well.

Add salt to taste, 1/8–1/4 teaspoon.

Mix 1/2 cup of the vegan cheese in.

Cut a rectangle in the pepper, removing the piece.

Cut out the membranes and seeds keeping the pepper intact.

Place pepper into a small baking dish.

Gently stuff the pepper with the mixture stretching the side's open and having a mound in the center. The entire pepper should be stuffed with the mixture.

Pat the 2 tablespoons of cheese over the exposed stuffing.

Bake 400 for 35 minutes. Cheese will begin to brown on the top.

Sweet Potato Enchiladas

I love the sweetness of the sweet potato in contrast to the spiciness of the green salsa. When I became dairy free, I tended to not cook anything in the beginning that I use to eat that had cheese. It was not until I discovered vegan cheese that I began to start doing that. These enchiladas are actually excellent even without vegan cheese. I have made them numerous times cheese less. I think it is because the sweet potatoes add such a nice flavor mixed with the green chilies and seasonings that you don't miss the cheese. I have written the recipe with the vegan cheese as an ingredient, but it can easily be omitted.

Prep Time: 15 minutes
Cook Time: 30 Minutes
Yield: 4 Servings

Ingredients:

2 sweet potatoes
1 can black beans
1 can green chilies (or 3 roasted and peeled ones)
1 red bell pepper diced
1 small yellow onion diced
2 garlic cloves minced

2 cups green salsa
12 corn tortillas
4 Tbsp. chopped cilantro
1 Tsp chili powder
1 Tsp cumin
1/2 Tsp salt
1/4 Tsp black pepper
1 bag of vegan shredded cheddar cheese (2 cups)

Instructions:

Pre heat oven 350° degrees Fahrenheit.

Peel and dice the sweet potatoes. Put in a sauce pot cover with cold water and bring to a boil.

Cook until sweet potatoes are tender and a fork can pierce easily about 12 minutes.

Drain and rinse the black beans or use 1 cups of homemade black beans. Place in a large bowl.

Add the cooked sweet potatoes, green chilies, diced onions, minced garlic, diced bell pepper, cilantro, chili powder, cumin, salt and pepper.

Mix well.

Put enough salsa to cover the bottom of a 9 x 13 inch baking dish.

Heat up the tortillas.

Put 3 tablespoons of sweet potato mix in the center of the tortilla and sprinkle with a tablespoon of the vegan cheddar cheese.

Roll the tortilla and put seam side down in the baking dish. Repeat with the rest of the tortillas filling each one, rolling and laying it in bottom of baking dish next to the prior one.

Pour remaining salsa over the enchiladas and sprinkle with 1 cup of the remaining cheese.

Bake for 30 minutes until done.

Tequila Orange Prawns

This is a quick, easy and delicious meal. I like to make this recipe with large prawns but you can substitute shrimp for it, just use more. I love the flavor of the fresh orange with the tequila. The tequila add flavor to the marinade and cooks off quickly when the prawns are in the pan. I also like to leave the last segment of the tail and tail fin on the prawns for presentation and for easy eating if you want to forgo the knife and fork! I like to pare this prawn dish with my quinoa Tabouli salad.

Prep Time: 5 Minutes
Cook Time: 3 Minutes
Yield: 1 Serving

Ingredients:

7 large prawns
Zest of one orange
Juice of one orange
3 Tablespoons good tequila
1 clove of garlic minced
1/4 teaspoon salt
Few grinds of pepper
1 Tablespoon coconut oil

Instructions:

Prep the prawns by peeling them and leaving the tail on.

With a paring knife, slice down the back 2/3 of the way through so that it butterflies and can stand up. Remove the vein, rinse and pat dry.

In a large zip bag add the orange zest, orange juice, tequila, minced garlic, teaspoon and pepper.

Mix well and add the shrimp.

Zip closed and put in the fridge for 1/2 to 1 hour, shaking the bag on occasion to make sure the prawns soak up the flavor.

In a small frying pan heat the coconut oil.

Once it is hot, place the prawns, butterflied side down curling the tail over it.

Cook until it starts to turn pink, about 2 minutes.

Sear each side quickly and the shrimp will turn orange and begin to curl into the letter C. Don't overcook.

Take out of the pan and plate.

These are even good room temp or chilled the next day.

Tuscan Pork

When I think of the flavors of Tuscany, I think of tomatoes, garlic, oregano and wine. This recipe blends those flavors together beautifully. The onions caramelize which adds a deep sweet note that blends nicely with the fire-roasted tomatoes.

The pork chops are browned and then nestled in the flavorful sauce as they gently cook. This is so good that it could also be done with chicken or the sauce alone over gluten free pasta.

Prep Time: 10 Minutes
Cook Time: 30-40 Minutes
Yields: 4 Servings

Ingredients:

4 pork chops, fat trimmed
1 tbsp. coconut oil
4 cloves of garlic, diced
1 can fire roasted tomatoes
1 large onion, finely diced
2 tsp oregano
1 tsp basil
1/2 tea salt
1/4 tea pepper
1/2 cup white wine

Instructions:

Heat a large skillet or Dutch oven on the stove over medium high heat.

Add the coconut oil and let it melt, coating the bottom of the pan.

Season the chops with a pinch of salt and pepper. Add to the pan and brown each side, about 3 minutes each side.

Remove chops from pan and set on plate to rest. (They are not done yet)

Reduce heat to medium-low, add onions. Stir onions and caramelize about 5 min they should be golden in color.

Add the tomatoes, garlic and spices and wine to the pan and stir to mix.

Bring the sauce up to a bubble and then nestle pork chops in mix and lower heat to med low

Cover and simmer until pork chops are done 15-20 minutes

Remove the pork chops and plate, spooning sauce over each one.

Vegan Ranch Dressing

I wanted a dairy free ranch dressing to go with a Cobb salad I had made. I knew that traditional ranch dressing had dairy. My final version tastes so good and you would not know it has coconut milk in it because of all of the fresh dill, and it tastes like traditional ranch dressing! This dressing also works great as a dip for veggies.

Prep Time: 15 Minutes
Yield: 2 cups

Ingredients:

1 cup mayo
1 1/4 cup coconut milk
3 tablespoons fresh chopped dill
3 cloves of garlic made into a paste with sea salt (use the flat side of your knife to do this)
1 1/2 teaspoons apple cider vinegar
3/4 teaspoon black pepper
1/8 teaspoon salt

Instructions:

Put all the ingredients into a blender and blend until smooth. (I actually put all the ingredients into a large glass jar and shake well.)

Veggie Herb and Egg Casserole

I have been so busy in the mornings that I wanted a quick and healthy breakfast full of protein and veggies. This recipe is delicious and you can adapt it to whatever kind of veggies you have on hand. I made a big casserole and it keeps well in the fridge and can be frozen. Healthy "fast" food!

You can substitute any veggies or herbs you have on hand and like. The veggies in the recipe where what I had on hand that day. Add chicken sausage for another variation.

It reheats well, is great at room temperature and you can cut into individual pieces, wrap with plastic wrap, drop it into a zip freezer bag and freeze. Now you have a fast and healthy meal on hand. Have it for dinner with a side salad or for brunch.

Prep Time: 15 Minutes
Cook Time: 35 Minutes
Yield: 6 Servings

Ingredients:

12 eggs
1 red bell pepper diced
1 yellow onion diced
2 cups of mushrooms sliced

2 tablespoons cilantro chopped
1/2 teaspoon salt
1/4 teaspoon fresh black pepper
1 tablespoons
1 teaspoon coconut oil divided

Instructions:

Preheat oven to 350° Fahrenheit

Beat the eggs in a large bowl.

Add the chopped cilantro, set aside.

Heat 1 tablespoon of coconut oil in a frying pan.

Sauté the diced bell pepper, diced onion and sliced mushrooms until tender.

Add the salt and pepper.

Cook about 5 minutes.

Turn off heat and let the mix cool to room temperature.

Oil the inside of a casserole dish with 1 teaspoon of coconut oil.

Put the cooled veggie mix on the bottom of the dish.

Pour the herb and egg mixture over and mix gently.

Bake in the oven for 35 minutes. The edges will brown up.

Let the casserole sit on the counter for 5-10 minutes before cutting.

White Bean Salad

Years ago I was at a Women's retreat and we were staying in a rustic lodge in the mountains of the Santa Cruz mountains in Northern California. We were blessed to have a chef prepare all of our meals for us. She made some very delicious food. One lunch she was grilling some fish and she made a white bean salad as the side dish. At first I took just a small portion because it did not look like anything special. I was so very, very wrong! It was indeed a special dish and I could not get enough of it.

The sweetness of the charred sweet onions mixing with the crunchiness of the cucumber along with the tang of the Dijon, red wine vinegar and capers made each mouthful divine! This is my version of that salad.

Prep Time: 10 Minutes
Cook Time: 10 Minutes
Yield: 2-3 Servings

Ingredients:

1 medium Vidalia or other sweet onion, cut into 1/4-inch-thick slices
3 tablespoons red wine vinegar
1 tablespoon olive oil

1/4 teaspoon salt
1/4 teaspoon freshly ground black pepper
1/4 teaspoon Dijon mustard
1 garlic clove, minced
1/2 cup chopped seeded peeled cucumber
1/4 cup chopped flat-leaf parsley
1 tablespoon capers
1 (15-ounce) can cannellini beans, rinsed and drained

Instructions:

Place onion slices on pre-heated grill. Grill 5 minutes on each side or until tender and charred. Cool and chop.

Combine vinegar, olive oil, salt, pepper, mustard and garlic clove in a large bowl, stirring with a whisk until emulsified.

Stir in the onion, cucumber, parsley, capers, and beans to vinegar mixture; toss to coat.

Zucchini Mini Muffins

Growing up we had a huge garden and tons of zucchini. When I was a young girl learning to cook, one of my go-to recipes was zucchini bread. I loved to make it and often put walnuts in it. Looking back I realize it was not really healthy because it was full of white flour and vegetable oil.

This recipe for mini muffins is easy to make and they turn out great. If you don't have a mini-muffin pan you can form them into small football-shaped pieces, put them on parchment paper on your baking sheet and cook them that way. When you do it this way the edges get nice and crunchy.

There is a lot of water in the squash so make sure to get it all squeezed out or these muffins will fall apart.

Prep Time: 15 Minutes
Cook Time: 20 Minutes
Yield: 12 Muffins

Ingredients:

1 tablespoon coconut oil
2 cups shredded zucchini (3-4 zucchinis)
2 eggs, beaten

1/2 medium onion, grated
1/2 cup gluten free breadcrumbs
1/2 teaspoon salt
1/4 teaspoon pepper

Instructions:

Preheat oven to 400° Fahrenheit.

Grease the mini muffin pan with the coconut oil.

Grate the zucchinis until you have 2 cups, no need to peel.

In a cheesecloth or kitchen towel, wring out all of the moisture.

In a medium bowl, combine all of the ingredients and season with salt and pepper to taste. Use your fingers to mix well.

Spoon some of the zucchini mixture in to the mini muffin pans.

Bake until they begin to brown about 20-25 minutes.

Take muffin tin out of the oven and let cool before removing.

Part 9: Master Checklists

Pantry Checklist

Grains

____ Arborio Rice
____ Black Rice
____ Brown Rice
____ Corn Meal/Polenta
____ Gluten Free Oats
____ Organic Masa Harina
____ Quinoa
____ Wild Rice

Nuts & Seeds

____ Brazil Nuts
____ Chia Seeds
____ Flax Seeds
____ Pecan Nuts
____ Pine Nuts
____ Raw Almonds
____ Raw Cashews
____ Walnuts

Legumes

___ Canned Beans
___ Cannellini Beans
___ Dried Beans
___ Garbanzo Beans
___ Kidney Beans
___ Lentils
___ Mung Beans
___ Pinto Beans

Basics

____ Agave
____ Black Pepper
____ Coconut Sugar
____ Corn Starch
____ Curry Paste
____ Himalayan Sea salt
____ Spices
____ Tamari or Coconut Aminos
____ Agave Ketchup
____ Balsamic Vinegar
____ Cocoa Powder
____ Coconut Oil
____ Dijon Mustard
____ Dried Cherries
____ Dried Herbs
____ Dried Raisins
____ Good Olive Oil
____ Good Vinegars
____ Herbal Tea
____ Maple Syrup
____ Medjool Dates
____ Sesame Oil
____ Vanilla

Staples

___ **Applesauce Organic**
___ **Rice Noodles**
___ **Anchovies**
___ **Canned Green Chilies**
___ **Capers**
___ **Coconut Milk**
___ **Dried Shitake Mushrooms**
___ **Fire Roasted Tomatoes**
___ **Gluten Free Pasta**
___ **Jar of Marinated Artichoke Hearts**
___ **Jar of Roasted Peppers**
___ **Rice Crackers**
___ **Rice Sheets**
___ **Stock (chicken, veggie and beef)**
___ **Tomato Paste**
___ **Tomato Sauce**
___ **Tuna**

Freezer Checklist

___ Bacon
___ Berries
___ Chicken Breast Tenders
___ Cooked Rice
___ Cooked Quinoa
___ Fish
___ Frozen Fruit
___ Frozen Veggies (variety)
___ Ginger, Whole
___ Gluten Free Bread
___ Grapes
___ Ground Beef
___ Ground Chicken
___ Herbs
___ Lemon Juice
___ Lemon Zest
___ Ripe Bananas
___ Sausages (chicken, beef or pork)
___ Shrimp
___ Stew Meat
___ Whole Chickens

Fridge Checklist

____ Apples
____ Baby spinach
____ Bell peppers
____ Berries
____ Broccoli
____ Capers
____ Carrots
____ Celery cucumber
____ Dijon mustard
____ Eggs
____ Fresh fruit
____ Fresh herbs
____ Fresh veggies
____ Garlic
____ Hummus
____ Lean ground beef
____ Lemons
____ Limes
____ Mayonnaise
____ Mushrooms
____ Nut butter

____ Onions
____ Organic agave ketchup
____ Potatoes
____ Roast chicken
____ Salad
____ Salsa
____ Shredded cabbage
____ Water

Shopping List

FRUIT AND VEGGIES

____ Baby spinach
____ Berries
____ Broccoli - 1-pound
____ Bunch green onions
____ Butter lettuce
____ Carrots - 8
____ Chard or kale
____ Cucumbers - 2
____ Fingerling or small potatoes - 1-pound
____ Gluten free oats
____ Head of garlic
____ Lemons - 5
____ Limes - 2
____ Melon
____ Mushrooms
____ Onions - 4
____ Papaya
____ Red bell peppers - 2
____ Salad green mix
____ Shredded purple cabbage
____ Spaghetti squash
____ Sweet potatoes - 3
____ Tomatoes - 6
____ Zucchini - 4

PROTEINS

____ Chicken breasts - 4 bone in
____ Ground beef - 2 pounds
____ Hard boiled eggs - dozen
____ Roast beef - 1 small or tri tip
____ Roast chicken - 1 whole
____ Tuna - 2 cans

Conversions and Substitutions

Substitutions for Items that have gluten:

Flour - use coconut flour, almond flour, amaranth flour
Bread - bread made from tapioca or rice as well as the flours above
Pasta - pasta made from rice, corn, garbanzo beans or quinoa
Soy Sauce - use coconut aminos or tamarind sauce

Substitutions for items that have dairy:

One-cup cow's milk: use one cup of the following: soy milk (plain),
Rice milk, fruit juice, water, coconut milk or hemp milk.

One-cup of yogurt: use one cup of the following: coconut yogurt, soy
Sour cream, unsweetened applesauce or fruit puree.

One-stick of butter:
8 tablespoons of coconut oil
8 tablespoons Vegan Buttery Spread
8 tablespoons Vegan Organic Shortening
8 tablespoons vegetable or olive oil
6 tablespoons unsweetened applesauce + 2 tablespoons on of the others in this list.

Breads:
Commercial Gluten Free Breads, rolls and wraps
Homemade Gluten Free breads, rolls, and wraps
Cauliflower breads, rolls, bagels and pizza crust
Bread Crumbs
Flax Meal
Crushed Nuts
Gluten Free Bread Crumbs
Potato Flakes

Buttermilk:
1 Tbsp. of vinegar to 1 cup of milk substitute of your choice

Cheese:
Nutritional Yeast
Zucchini Cheese
Plant based cheese
Cashew Cream

Cream, condensed and evaporated milks:
Coconut milk creamers
Full fat coconut milk
Coconut Cream
Homemade Versions

Eggs:

Flax Egg: Begin with whole, raw flax seeds and grind them fresh. One
Egg equals: 1 tablespoon flax meal plus 3 tablespoons water. Add the
Ground flax seed to the water and mix well with a fork or mini whisk.
Refrigerate for 15 minutes and up to an hour for the egg to set up properly. The ground flax seed forms a sticky goo that is similar to egg
Whites.

Chia Egg: Using a food processor, spice grinder, or mortar & pestle, grind 1 tablespoon of chia seeds. Soak the ground meal of chia seeds in
3 Tablespoons of warm water for 5 minutes. The seeds will expand and turn into a goopy texture similar to an egg. Chia seeds are gluten-free and grain-free, high in omega-3 fatty acids and are an
Excellent source of magnesium.

Slurry Binder: For this you can use arrowroot powder, potato or gluten free cornstarch. Mix 2 tablespoons of one of those with 2-3 tablespoons water and mix well before adding to your sauce or other items.

Mashed Fruit Binder: When you are baking something like cookies or sweeter tasting breads you can mash up bananas (1 small) or use ¼ cup of fruit puree. Not only will it give you the moisture of an egg it will naturally sweeten without using any added sugar. A ¼ cup of applesauce works great here too.

Flour Substitutes:
Amaranth Flour
Arrowroot Flour
Brown Rice Flour
Buckwheat Flour
Chia Flour
Chickpea Flour
Corn Flour
Cornmeal
Hemp Flour
Lupin Flour
Maize Flour
Millet Flour
Oat Flour-from certified oats
Potato Flour
Potato Starch Flour
Quinoa Flour
Sorghum Flour
Tapioca Flour
Teff Flour
White Rice Flour
Commercial Flour Blends
Homemade Flour Blends

Milk:
Almond Milk
Cashew Milk
Coconut Milk Beverages
Coconut Milk
Hemp Milk
Oat Milk
Rice Milk

Pasta:
Gluten Free Pasta
Spaghetti Squash
Zucchini Noodles

Sour cream and cream cheese:
Commercial substitutes using coconut milk
Plant based cream cheese

Soy Sauce:
Coconut Aminos
Gluten Free Soy Sauce
Tamari Sauce

Sugar Substitutes:
Stevia
Agave Nectar
Coconut Palm Sugar
Coconut Nectar
Honey
Molasses
Real Maple Syrup
Brown Rice syrup
Rapadura or Sucanat
Yacón Syrup
No Sugar added mashed fruit (for baking)

Yogurt:
Coconut milk yogurt
Almond yogurt
Chia Seed Yogurt
Coconut milk with grass fed gelatin

Whipped Cream:
Commercial substitutes
Coconut Cream Whipped

About The Author

Michelle E. DeBerge is a Foodie, Chef, Professional Life Coach, Motivational Speaker, America's Leading Life Redesign Expert, and Bestselling Author.

She uses her own experience of a serious health scare, her recovery, her discovery and study with some of the world's top experts in nutrition, diet and health, to form the foundation for her health and wellness programs.

Michelle's ultimate mission: To help you achieve more success, achieve your dreams and design the healthy lifestyle you desire for the long term.

She has rewritten her cookbooks to create her recipes gluten, sugar, dairy free. They have bold flavor, international flair and are quick and easy. Since she struggled physically for so many years, it is her passion to help others be healthy and do it with ease and grace.

Michelle's authenticity in identifying with the struggles that so many face has been a key factor in Michelle's success. She inspires personal growth and motivates people to redesign and renew their lives. She blends spirituality, experience, lifestyle, health, wellness and coaching together to create unique programs for her clients and audience.

She has helped guide her clients over the past 15 years to great success through a proven method of training, daily support and more. Using a time-honored, holistic approach that acknowledges the contributions of mind, body and spirit.

Websites:

www.glutensugardairyfree.com

www.lifecoach-usa.com

Contact:

michelle@michelledeberge.com

Reviewers

Dr John DeWitt

Dr. DeWitt is a Vanderbilt University graduate who earned a full athletic scholarship after his first semester. He went on to become the starting defensive end for the next four years and was awarded The Wade Looney Award for outstanding work ethic. He continued his football career with the NFL Houston Oilers, NFL Europe Champion Scottish Claymores, Montreal Alouettes of the CFL, San Francisco Demons of the XFL, and several teams in the AFL including three seasons with the LA Avengers.

After retiring from football, Dr. DeWitt earned his Doctor of Chiropractic degree from Los Angeles Chiropractic College. He is practicing in Orange County, at Bergman Family Chiropractic, specializing in personal injury cases and corrective chiropractic care.

He is an active volunteer for the Assistance League of Newport-Mesa, the Lili Claire Foundation and supporter of Boys Town of California. He can be seen on the Healthy OC segment of the Real OC on KOCE hosted by Heidi Cortese.

Dr DeWitt is a certified advanced sports nutrition specialist. He has over 10 years of nutritional counseling and exercise coaching.
drjohndewitt.com
theballersite.com
stopelbowinjuries.com

Kate and Justin Stellman

Kate and Justin Stellman are the founders and the radio show hosts of Extreme Health Radio.

Extreme Health Radio is a wildly popular online radio show inviting people around the globe to invest in themselves physically, spiritually and emotionally.

Hosts Justin and Kate Stellman provide ever-green and life changing information from highly acclaimed doctors, scientists, healers and authors. Start your journey to discover the best version of yourself today!

http://www.extremehealthradio.com/gsdf

Resources

David Zivot- Founder GrainStorm Heritage Baking Company-VP of Operations for Goodlife Magazine

Michael Specter, The New Yorker
Michael Specter, staff writer at *The New Yorker*, he has twice received the Global Health Council's annual Excellence in Media Award. He received the 2002 AAAS Science Journalism Award. His piece "Against the Grain" won a 2015 James Beard Award in the Food and Health category.

Dr. David Perlmutter
David Perlmutter, MD, FACN, ABIHM is a Board-Certified Neurologist and Fellow of the American College of Nutrition. He has contributed extensively to the world medical literature with publications appearing in The Journal of Neurosurgery, The Southern Medical Journal, Journal of Applied Nutrition, and Archives of Neurology. Dr. David Perlmutter is recognized internationally as a leader in the field of nutritional influences in neurological disorders. Dr. Perlmutter was the recipient of the National Nutritional Foods Association Clinician of the Year Award and was awarded the Humanitarian of the Year award from the American College of Nutrition.

The cornerstone of Dr. Perlmutter's unique approach to neurological disorders is founded in the principles of preventive medicine. He has brought to the public awareness a rich understanding that challenging brain problems including Alzheimer's disease, other forms of dementia, depression, and ADHD may very well be prevented with lifestyle changes including a gluten free, low carbohydrate, higher fat diet coupled with aerobic exercise.

Professor Peter Gibson

Peter is Professor and Director of Gastroenterology at The Alfred and Monash University, He is a Past-President of the Gastroenterological Society of Australia. From a background of research in epithelial cell biology, he now runs a large program of translational research and has active clinical interests in inflammatory bowel disease, coeliac disease and irritable bowel syndrome. A major focus of his work is the use of diet to control gut symptoms and influence outcomes in chronic intestinal conditions.

Sébastien Noël-

Due to health problems since his childhood Mr. Noel has developed a healthy way of eating that help alleviate his symptoms. He has done years of research to find out the healthiest way to eat for his health issues

Dr. David Reuben, M. D., is a Physician and Surgeon with a specialty in Psychiatry. After internship and residency he served as a Medical Officer with the U.S. Air Force before establishing his own medical offices. He has practiced medicine in Illinois, and California.
His other eight books have revolutionized scientific concepts of good health in many ways. For example, The Save-Your-Life Diet™ transformed the dietary habits in America as well as in many countries around the world.

David Schardt is Senior Nutritionist for NutritionAction.com®. Schardt has been writing about nutrition for the general public and for professionals for more than 25 years. His reports on nutrition and dietary supplements are featured in Nutrition Action Healthletter. He helped to write and edit the landmark Surgeon General's Report on Nutrition and Health. His book Eating Leaner and Lighter, published by Warner Books, was recommended for sensible nutrition by the USDA's Food and Nutrition Information Center.

He has been featured on numerous television and radio programs and is widely quoted in the print media, especially on the subject of dietary supplements. David has graduate degrees in nutrition and biochemistry from Oregon State University and graduate study and research experience with Cornell University's Division of Nutritional Sciences.

Tori Avery- Is a foodie and an experienced home cook who has learned, over the years, how to cook dishes from all over the world. Through her own research, she has found the healthiest way to cook and live.

Carl H. Johnson, Ph.D.

Stevenson Professor of Biological Sciences, Professor of Biological Sciences, Professor of Molecular Physiology and Biophysics Vanderbilt University. He specializes in Cellular and Molecular Biology of Biological Clocks.

Jeanne Segal, Ph.D., has been helping individuals and families for over 40 years as an innovator in the fields of emotional intelligence, holistic health, attachment, stress reduction, and relationships. She has written five books, which have been published in 13 languages.

Lawrence Robinson, Editor, is a freelance writer with over ten years experience working for print and online publications, covering a wide range of subjects in the health and fitness fields. He is also a published author and has edited several books on psychology.

Professor Carlo Leifert

Res Dev Prof of Ecological Agriculture

Carlo was appointed as Research Development Professor for Ecological Agriculture at Newcastle University

Annie B. Bond is a green-living advocate, author, editor, entrepreneur, and consultant. She is currently the editor-in-chief of *The Wellness Wire*. Bond has written five books on green living and was named "the foremost expert on green living" by *Body & Soul* magazine.

The Macrobiotics Guide- a webpage guide, with articles and tools to lead the macrobiotic life
http://www.macrobiotics.co.uk/

Marije Hamaker-at the end of what sugar does to the body

Visit Our Site:
www.glutensugardairyfree.com

Find Out More About The GSDF 8 Week Companion Course

www.glutensugardairyfree.com/companion-course

This course goes in depth into all 8 of the main sections of the book.

- Really understand gluten, sugar and dairy, what it does to the body and how to avoid it.
- Learn to look at food differently and set healthy goals.
- Learn how to choose healthy foods, understand GMO's and other toxins.
- Understand your bodies triggers, how to set yourself up for success and be empowered.
- Learn everything you need to have in a GSDF household and kitchen for success.
- The inside tricks and tips to making healthy GSDF meals in minutes.
- Learn to master conversions and substations of standard recipes into GSDF ones with ease.
- Learn easy recipes, how to create delicious meal plans and feed your family on the fly.
- Live Q&A with the author every class!! Personal Support for your success.

Visit Our Site:
www.glutensugardairyfree.com

Printed in Great Britain
by Amazon.co.uk, Ltd.,
Marston Gate.